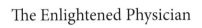

The Enlightened Physician

The Enlightened Physician

Achille-Cléophas Flaubert, 1784–1846

Geoffrey Wall

Peter Lang Oxford

First published in 2013 by

Peter Lang Ltd
International Academic Publishers
52 St Giles, Oxford
Oxfordshire OX1 3LU
United Kingdom

www.peterlang.com

Geoffrey Wall has asserted his right under the Copyright, Designs
and Patents Act of 1988 to be identified as the Author of this Work.

© Peter Lang Ltd 2013

A catalogue record for this book is available from the British Library

ISBN 978-1-906165-47-5

COVER ILLUSTRATION:

Joanna Neborsky

Every effort has been made to trace copyright holders and to obtain their permission
for the use of copyright material. The publisher apologises for any errors or omissions
and would be grateful for notification of any corrections that should be incorporated
in future reprints or editions of this book.

Printed in the United Kingdom by TJ International

The writing of cultural descriptions is properly experimental
and ethical. […] It looks obliquely at all collective arrangements.
What are these ceremonies and why should we take part in them?
What are these professions and why should we make money
out of them?

James Clifford, *Writing Culture* (1986)

Contents

viii

Notes on the Text

A Note On Translations

All translations, unless otherwise attributed, are by the author.

The French Revolutionary Calendar

The French Revolutionary calendar was a distinctive and contentious feature of the radical political culture of the 1790s. In October 1793, at a time of war and social crisis, it was decreed by the Convention that the old Gregorian calendar was to be replaced by a properly republican calendar, designed to celebrate the fact that 'a new era in human history had begun following the overthrow of Louis XVI'.* True to the larger purpose of de-Christianisation, the months were renamed, according to reason and nature, drawing upon the seasonal round of the months. Because the republican year began on 22 September, none of the twelve newly named months coincided fully with any of the old months.

> Vendémiare: the month of vintage
> Brumaire: the month of fog
> Frimaire: the month of frost

---

* C. Jones, *The Longman Companion to the French Revolution*. London: Longman, 1988, 428.

Nivôse: the month of snow
Pluviôse: the month of rain
Ventôse: the month of wind
Germinal: the month of germination
Floréal: the month of flowering
Prairial: the month of meadows
Messidor: the month of harvest
Thermidor: the month of heat
Fructidor: the month of fruit

The new calendar remained in use, at least in official circles, until Napoleon abolished it in December 1806. In everyday life, apart from the crisis years of 1793–4 when it was prudent to use only the new calendar, the old and the new were used alongside each other, according to one's current political disposition.

Apart from the poetic ingenuity of the new names for the months, these names often figure prominently in the unfolding story of the revolution. They were used to designate moments of national crisis. Two such examples stand out. The fall of Robespierre and his faction in July 1793 is referred to as Thermidor. Napoleon's coup d'état in November 1799 is known as the Eighteenth Brumaire.

A Note on the Medical Dissertation of Achille-Cléophas Flaubert

THE AUTHOR'S TRANSLATION of the full text of Achille-Cléophas Flaubert's medical dissertation of 1811 is available online at no extra cost. It can be downloaded in pdf format at www.peterlang.com from the page for *The Enlightened Physician*.

This dissertation is of compelling interest as a document of the intellectual biography of an individual physician. It testifies, in its vividly detailed clinical observations, to exceptional qualities of compassion and empathy. These qualities are allied in this instance to an exemplary commitment to the larger social and ethical values of enlightenment science. If, in a spirit of adventure, you wish to grasp something of the traumatic experience of undergoing a surgical operation in the years before the invention of anaesthetic, this document will satisfy even the most demanding historical imagination. Here is the world of the urban hospital, in the very early years of modern scientific medicine. Read, reflect and give thanks.

Preface: Children of Napoleon

WHAT DID IT MEAN to be an enlightened physician, in the very early years of the nineteenth century? This book offers one kind of answer to that question. It takes the form of a narrative of the life of one eminently enlightened physician, in an age when science and religion had not yet settled into their current mode of irritable coexistence. This book is also, along the way, an informal group portrait of a generation of the medical profession, caught at the time just before the various discoveries that have made treatment both effective and endurable. Any list of those discoveries would include at least anesthetic, antisepsis, scientific pharmacology and the germ theory of infection.

The enlightened physician of my title is Achille-Cléophas Flaubert. In the eyes of his contemporaries, he was almost a great man. It would have distressed him profoundly, had he been told that he would only be remembered as the father of that scandalous bourgeois-baiting scribbler, his younger son, Gustave Flaubert. The physician of his generation was acclaimed, from within the profession and without, as the priest of humanity. He was a man of vision and energy, a man with a purity of purpose who had renounced the destructive political passions that led the men of 1789 to disaster in the name of their ideals. In his more grandiose moments, the enlightened physician might claim to be that elusive, necessary individual, the bourgeois hero.

That is certainly the message of the following eloquent testimonial to the ideal, written by Achille-Cléophas's friend and colleague. I quote from the manuscript notebook in which that colleague recorded his general moral reflections on a lifetime of medical practice.

A truly enlightened physician, dedicated to and worthy of the lofty mission which he pursues in this world, such a man will not blindly follow the fashion of the hour or espouse those political passions which so divide our society. The physician sees his fellow creatures on their bed of pain, far from the scenes of the fashionable world. The most afflicted and the most wretched, they are those that interest him the most. The physical and moral infirmities of the human race are perpetually before his gaze. Leaving the palatial dwelling of the rich, he enters the damp hovel of the poor, and there in both places he finds the same suffering creature, begging for his help. To their well-being he has consecrated his whole life. In his intimate contact with every class of society, he is ideally placed to observe, to know and to judge the human race, and to value it at its true worth. It does not in general present its most appealing side to him. He studies it from too close by; and though he may shed some pleasant illusions in the process, he can at least see the object as it really is. Calm in the midst of the chaos all around him, he simply deplores the unhappy consequences for the losers, moderates the anger or the self-importance of the victorious, laments subsequent misfortunes and disasters and endeavours to remedy them as far as it lies within his power. Minister of peace and unity between men who have confided in him all that they hold most dear, their lives and often their honour, he must simply console or cure them of their ailments, and if it is given to him to have any influence over them he will use it to moderate their passions, to guide them towards reason, justice and tolerance, towards all that he believes will be most useful for them and best for the country. As for the physician himself, his only legitimate ambition is to excel by virtue of his altruism, by the self-abnegation he displays in the midst of those epidemics that devastate whole cities, by his devotion and his courage in picking up or succouring the wounded on the field of battle; by his charity, by his severity in judging vice and his indulgence in judging the weaknesses of the human race. Such should be, in my opinion, the character, the duty and the veritable patriotism of the physician.[1]

It will be amusing and instructive, along the way, to recall this high vision of saintly benevolence as it unravels, in the medium of biographical narrative time, under the action of all the miscellaneously tragicomic forces that shape a life.

Where does a biography begin? Is it with an idealised array of ancestors? With the material realities of childhood? Or with adult memories of the early years? Researching my earlier biography of Gustave Flaubert in 1998, I soon renounced the idea of finding that elusively singular beginning. I strayed from the path, drawn back in time, down into ever-earlier layers of Flaubert family history. In particular, I was intrigued by a story from the 1860s that dealt with an episode from the childhood of Gustave's father in the 1790s. I found the story recorded in that compendium of nineteenth-century Parisian salon gossip, the Goncourts' *Journal*.

Here it is, as told to them by their forty-two-year-old dinner guest Gustave Flaubert. It forms part of the journal entry for 26 January 1863.

> Flaubert told me, one evening recently, that his paternal grandfather, a doctor of the old school, having wept in an inn while reading in a newspaper of the execution of Louis XIV, arrested and about to be sent to the Revolutionary Tribunal in Paris, was saved by his own son, then aged seven, to whom his mother had taught a pathetic speech, which he delivered with great success to the Société populaire in Nogent-sur-Seine.[2]

It caught my eye, that climactic scene, with the child delivering his 'pathetic speech'. Here was a thing that might define a life, permeating the subsequent family history, encapsulating their painful collective memory of the revolution. In the face of oppression, it testified to the individual redemptive powers of language. Here was my elusive biographical beginning.

Even so, there was something odd about this episode. The story was simply too good to be true. So why had that story survived? What was it saying about the mid-century memory of the Revolution? Fortuitously preserved, this precious piece of oral tradition exists only in this meagre version. There is no mention of it in the official twenty-page obituary memoir of Flaubert's father, published in 1847. This was a significant silence, a minor family secret, asking to be gently unfolded.

Whatever else it might be, this was a compelling, diminutive life-or-death story. It had all the ingredients of popular romantic fiction: the injustice, the mortal distress, the child-hero, the surprise happy ending. I wondered why it had been kept quiet. I was keen to establish which bits were true. I promised myself that I would one day try to answer these questions. After Gustave, I would write the life of his father.

This book, a narrative biography of the life of Achille-Cléophas Flaubert, has emerged from the compacted historical memory that is preserved in the Goncourt *Journal*. This book is also the culmination of a larger Flaubert project that began in 1986, the year that I embarked on my translation of *Madame Bovary*. My translation of that novel led to a further translation, a selection of Flaubert's letters, published in 1996. That translation in turn led to a biography of Gustave Flaubert, published in 2001. These four books, two translations and two biographies, are linked by the conviction that literary translation and biography are complementary modes of knowledge.

Though mothers and wives, sisters and daughters will all play their part, this book is primarily a story of fathers and sons. The life of Achille-Cléophas unfolds from 1784 to 1846. Around that central panel we follow the history of three Flaubert generations. This is a history that spans a hundred years, from the 1760s to the 1860s, from the Ancien Régime to the railway age, a biography gleefully stretched across time and space. In that adventurous spirit, there will be several well-organised excursions along the way. Suitably clad and equipped, we shall visit cesspools, convents, dissection rooms, textile factories, shopping arcades, mortuaries, courtrooms, prison yards, museums, botanical gardens, hospital wards and country houses. We shall linger instructively over some of the major novelties of the age, the guillotine, the gaslight, the spinning jenny and the steam engine, devices that changed the very fabric of everyday life. Our subject, Achille-Cléophas, lived through interesting times. The strange things happening all around him will figure prominently. And because he witnesses much more than he can properly understand, he will be the focal point for an ironic narrative of a tumultuous modernity.

I shall argue, along the way, that even the most insolently aspiring and triumphantly self-made modern individual remains a creature of history, enacting their idiosyncratic version of the larger collective history of their class, their generation, and their gender. Idiosyncratic: that emphasis is vital. It points to that trans-historical 'family plot', according to which individual protagonists assert their own peculiar place in a line of succession defined by a shared family name. To carry that family name, to be a Flaubert, that was a serious task. To also become yourself, to do it better or to do it differently, that was a task even more demanding. This tangled play of freedom and necessity, this double history, must be the proper territory of the biographer.

Achille-Cléophas survived Robespierre and the Terror; he thrived under Napoleon. Then, in spite of his cumbersome political opinions, his imprudent atheism and his relative youth, he was appointed to high professional office in the very month that the House of Bourbon was restored to the throne of France. To write such a life is to explore the curiously complicated moral history of that insurgent, de-Christianised generation that came of age in the years between Austerlitz and Waterloo. The children of Voltaire and Napoleon, they had grown up as the citizens of a republic that mutated into an empire. Consequently, they had much to ponder in the late summer of 1815, finding themselves, so unexpectedly, the reluctant subjects of an aggressively conservative monarchy that was intent on imposing the curious fiction that the Revolution had not happened.

Acknowledgements

M Y THANKS TO ALL who have so generously given their individual advice and support: Gianna Chadwick, Jean-Pierre Chaline, Timothy Chesters, Alan Forrest, Yvan Leclerc, David Moody, Mary Orr, Sara Perren, Ronen Steinberg, Robert Tombs and Tim Unwin.

My special thanks to Malcolm Colledge, who was initially my collaborator on this project. He helped greatly to get it off the ground, though he bears no responsibility for its ultimate air-worthiness. A congenial companion in the archives, his comprehensive knowledge of medical history, his eye for clinical detail and his generous practical support have all made this a much better book.

Equal thanks to all those benevolent and hospitable guardians of the archive, the public institutions of French culture: the Société Archaéologique de Sens, the Bibliothèque de l'Académie nationale de médecine in Paris, and the Musée Flaubert et d'histoire de la médecine in Rouen.

My thanks to the Leverhulme Trust for a Research Fellowship in 2007.

My thanks to Faber and Faber, for permission to incorporate three brief passages, duly modified by further research, from my biography of Gustave Flaubert published in 2001.

1

Ancien Régime

An uncommon cheerfulness prevailed everywhere, among the friends of
the Revolution.
— BENJAMIN RUSH, *Medical Inquiries and Observations* (1805)

IN A COUNTRY VILLAGE on a bend of the river Seine, far from the
sea, in the soon-to-be-abolished province of Champagne, a child is
born on 14 November 1784, into a modest, provincial artisan family
of veterinary surgeons and blacksmiths. His mother gives birth to him,
her first child, at the sensible age of twenty-seven, in the house where
she herself was born. Prudently pious, the parents have the infant chris-
tened some hours before the end of his first day in the world. He is called
Achille-Cléophas Flaubert.

Four years and eight months after this perfectly inconspicuous domes-
tic event, the Revolution will embark on the reinvention of time, space and
God. Within twenty years there will be a new hierarchy based on property,
education and energy. Scornfully or wistfully, according to taste, people
will speak of 'the days of the seigneurs', a phrase that endured in popular
memory.[1] The events of the Revolution will encroach upon, though they
will scarcely erase, the stubborn old hierarchy of birth and privilege. For
the moment though, continuity seems to be written into the everyday
order of things. Despite the murmurings of a dissident philosophical
elite, this is still a world divided into three legally distinct social orders.

The ill-fated class structure of pre-revolutionary France can be
briskly described. One per cent of the population are of noble status.
They number around 250,000, and they own around 25 per cent of the

land.[2] All this seductive aristocratic elegance is ravenously expensive; the institutional piety that secures social cohesion is almost equally costly. To add to the burdens already laid upon the backs of the tax-paying population, the clergy, around 170,000 in number, own a further 10 per cent of the land.[3]

Achille-Cléophas Flaubert: this child's name, in its separate parts, is a nice conjunction of the classical, the biblical and the solidly regional. 'Achille' was not chosen for any fanciful heroic radiance. It pointed prosaically to the child's godfather, Louis Achille Petel, one of a local dynasty of *maîtres de postes* and *aubergistes*. Both Louis Petel and his wife signed the parish register on that short November day. The fact of their literacy suggests that the parents of the newborn were well connected, linked to the prosperous and educated local elite, men and women of substance. 'Cléophas' was the pious choice. It was the name of one of the two disciples to whom the risen Lord appeared at Emmaeus. 'Cléophas' might become a liability, once the de-Christianisation campaigns of the early 1790s began to bite. Minor officials will write it down as 'Cléopâtre' in their documents.

The family name, Flaubert, was the child's most tangible asset in a world where sons still followed, mostly, in the footsteps of their fathers. A good name was a piece of solid cultural capital, 'a durable network of more or less institutionalized relationships of mutual acquaintance and recognition', an intangible patrimony of 'knowledge needed to succeed'.[4] In good families, always a nicely resonant phrase, such matters were tacitly understood. On the larger stage, in the modern drama of individual ambition, patronage remained a decisive force. The public realm would soon be open to talent. Yet talent would never be a purely rational quantity, something that could be measured by exam results. Talent would depend for its realisation on affective social bonds closely modelled on those of father and son.

This benign patriarchal continuity of the early years did not last. Consider the fact that, when Achille-Cléophas was eight years old, they executed the king. When he was nine they put his father in prison. When he was eleven, he embarked on an Enlightenment education in a Jacobin town where Christianity had been abolished and the churches were locked. When he was nineteen he arrived in Paris, a medical student, just as General Bonaparte, now First Consul, adopted the more regal title of Napoleon. When he was thirty-one, in the week of the battle of Waterloo, he was appointed chief surgeon in the main hospital of the great textile city of Rouen. Lecturing on physiology, he expounded Bichat's new map of the human body, a map from which the ancient province of the soul had been discreetly erased. From the age of nine, until the age of thirty-one, Achille-Cléophas lived in a nation at war.

Contemplating only the first thirty years of this man's life, we shall observe what Marx described, in another context, as 'uninterrupted disturbance of all social conditions, everlasting uncertainty and agitation'.[5] There was indeed the restless moral energy of modernity at work in this family history. But there was also a striking continuity, even across the events of the 1790s. Back in the 1770s this talented provincial family was already connected, through education, and through their qualifications, to the wider national life, although under the guild system they were confined, professionally, to their province of origin. There was, inevitably, a certain tension between those soon-to-be abolished particularisms and the new emphasis on a national Republican identity. There were vivid, modern, metropolitan interludes in this larger family history, yet the underlying pattern of small-town life persisted.

To UNDERSTAND THE CONTINUITIES in this chronicle of social advancement, we shall now reach further back into that family history. In 1784, when Achille-Cléophas was born, the Flaubert family had long been established in the Anglure region of the north-eastern province of Champagne. Nearly one hundred years previously, there had been a Flaubert who, in 1696, already had his coat of arms with *flammes d'or*. The flames in that coat of arms signified the giant scalpel that was the formidable tool of the animal-surgical trade. Achille-Cléophas's immediate paternal ancestors came from Bagneux, a village in the valley of the river Aube, one of the four main tributaries of the Seine. Bagneux was a small village that sat in the shadow of a large chateau. The silhouette of the two great towers, an everyday lesson in the splendours of hierarchy, rose above the trees on the island in the middle of the river Aube.

In the village of Bagneux the breeding of horses was a speciality. The care of horses was the Flaubert family business. In winter a regiment of cavalry was quartered in the town. A cavalry sergeant stood as godfather to a Flaubert in 1722. Flaubert men had also been blacksmiths only two generations before Achille-Cléophas, though there had long been Flaubert

relations who were qualified vets and men of position in the local administration. In the later years of the eighteenth century, this was a family on
the way up. In the course of three generations they would evolve rapidly,
from blacksmith to vet, and then from vet to doctor. They would also
migrate from village to town and from town to city.

Nicolas Flaubert, father of Achille-Cléophas, was born in 1754. He
was the second of three sons. All three Flaubert siblings received the
same costly education and eventually practised the same profession of
veterinary medicine. At the age of twenty-one in November 1775, Nicolas
enrolled in the recently established Royal Veterinary School at Alfort, just
south of Paris. In doing so he was following in the footsteps of his older
brother, Jean-Baptiste. Nicolas now had a five-year professional training
ahead of him, all to be paid for, once again, by his father. The veterinary
training at Alfort was expensive: 120 livres per year for board, sixty livres
for the uniform and another sixty livres for books, scalpels and a leather
apron. It was presumably a sound investment. Only a confidently prosperous blacksmith would have the money to bestow such an education
on all three of his sons.

Founded only nine years previously, in 1766, Alfort was the first veterinary school to be established in Europe. This initiative was prompted
by progressive physiocrat doctrine on the subject of national wealth in
land. State investment in the amelioration of agriculture was decreed to
be money well spent. Improvements to the medical care of farm animals
were imperative. The Alfort school was thus located in a suitably imposing set of buildings, recently purchased by the state from its aristocratic
owners. We may describe the fabric of the school in some detail, drawing on a description published in 1781, the year after Nicolas graduated.

Half a day's journey south east of Paris, the Alfort school was housed
in a large chateau set in extensive parkland, amid ploughed fields, at the
confluence of the Seine and the Marne. The school was a place of regal
splendour. The student newly arrived from some provincial town had
probably never seen anything like it before. The main entrance had a
set of magnificently elaborate wrought-iron gates manned by a Swiss
Guard in royal livery. Beyond the gates one entered a spacious courtyard
lined with trees. There was a large chapel, the interior painted to look
like marble. In the teaching block there was a cabinet of curiosities, miscellaneous objects designed to stimulate an interest in natural history.
Students remembered particularly the prize exhibit, a life-size anatomy

model of a man, 'terrible and menacing' and 'most artistically executed in wax'. There was also a library and then, just beyond the library, a big dissection room with a dozen large oak tables and special stone floors to drain away body fluids. The facilities included a stable block, a forge and a botanical garden for herbal remedies.

The decorative scheme in the main hall, *la salle des concours*, displayed the familiar images and emblems of the veterinary art: utensils for the stable, tools for the forge, a cow's head neatly dissected, an array of syringes, a collection of surgical instruments, and then a botanical emblem with a cluster of flowers tastefully arranged. Two stone tablets with Latin inscriptions, one above each door, completed the effect. They read *Dii patrii, purgamus agros, purgamus agrestes, Vos mala de nostris pellite limitibus* ('Gods of our fathers, drive evil away, make fertile our fields, abundant our flocks'). By memorising these lines, taken from the elegies of Tibullus, the ambitious student might hope one day to hold his own in circles where the elite game of Latin quotation was played out. Beyond the *salle de concours* and its poetic intimations of future cultural capital, there was the prosaic actuality of a pharmacy: a suite of laboratories where medicines were prepared. This room had a range of cupboards with porcelain jars for ingredients. Here the ailing poor sometimes came for their medicines.[6]

The ethos at Alfort was distinctly strenuous. Students enjoyed – and often endured – a strong *esprit de corps*. They were subject to a rigorous military code of discipline and they wore a costly uniform, sixty-livres-worth of Ancien Régime magnificence. The regulations specified a royal blue tunic with six gilded brass buttons all embossed with the fleur-de-lys and inscribed École royale Vétérinaire. It was compulsory to wear this uniform at all times when outside the school; though in case they should entertain ideas beyond their station, students were forbidden to carry swords. This privilege was reserved for the staff. In this place, under these conditions, in his new uniform, a young man would realise within a few hours that he was going to be part of something important.[7]

The programme of study at Alfort in the 1770s included anatomy, physiology, hygiene, artistic anatomy, pharmacy and forge work.[8] This ambitious union of theory and practice provoked conflict with some of the vested interests of the day. There was resistance from the powerful corporation of blacksmiths, wary of all such encroachments upon their particular sphere. Equally, there was suspicion among the physicians and the surgeons. In the 1780s, after Nicolas had graduated, instruction was further transformed. Medical reformers took over, inspired the creation of new positions and initiated advanced research. Lack of funds, later in that decade, reduced the scientific content of instruction, but the ideal of a unified human and animal medicine was not abandoned.[9]

The Alfort class of 1775 received a technical, scientific education at the highest level. Even so, under Bourgelat, its founding director, Alfort was not a happy ship in the early years. His temper soured by the agonies of gout, Bourgelat exercised a 'violent despotism'.[10] Independence and originality were suppressed in teachers and students alike. None of the staff published anything during his tenure, because the director ruthlessly plagiarised their work. Many tutors were driven out, or they simply left the school, unable to bear his domineering style.[11] After the death of Bourgelat in 1779, Alfort was renewed, from above, by a generation of progressive medical reformers.

I have located three surviving objects from Alfort: a statue, a book and a document. Each of these objects can tell us a great deal, both about Nicolas's individual experience of Alfort and about the larger medical world in the years before 1789. The statue is an anatomy model. The book is a flora compiled by Nicolas during his student years. The document is the *brevet*, the patent, awarded to the graduating student in the name of Louis XVI.

The anatomy model was the work of Honoré Fragonard (1732–1799), the cousin and the contemporary of the famous painter. Trained as a surgeon, Fragonard was recruited to be the first professor of anatomy at Alfort. An advocate of so-called natural anatomy, he used the traditional techniques of preserving bodies, either in alcohol or by desiccation. Alongside thousands of routine preparations intended for teaching anatomy, Fragonard created an elaborate symbolic *écorché* – literally a flayed body – entitled 'The Horseman of the Apocalypse'. It was an evocation of the famous engraving by Dürer. The work of five years, from 1766 to 1771, it shows – or rather it *is* – a man riding on a galloping horse. Both horse and rider have been stripped of skin and muscles. The nerves and the arteries are exposed. To complete the symbolism, the two main figures of man and horse are accompanied by a troop of human foetuses riding on the backs of flayed sheep.

It is worth emphasising that Fragonard's perfectly macabre creation is only a slightly more extravagant version of images and practices that were the familiar medical currency of the day. In the social practice of anatomy, art and science were not yet distinct. Anatomy was not yet regarded as merely a form of scientific research. It was the opportunity for a symbolic morality tale on the theme of death. In the next generation, when Achille-Cléophas received *his* medical training, the fanciful conjunction represented by Fragonard's *écorché* was slowly dissolving in favour of the more rational practice of the dissection of real corpses.

Let us turn from the *écorché* to the book. In May 1778, during the third year of his studies, Nicolas Flaubert compiled a large flora, a collection of dried plants arranged to illustrate the principles of taxonomy. A richly decorative and surprisingly large object, the book testifies to its author's declared affiliation to the cultural and scientific elite of the day. Preserved in the municipal museum in Rouen, the flora is a 726-page folio volume, bound in calfskin, embossed with the fleur-de-lys in gold at its four corners, along with the royal coat of arms on the boards. The spine is inscribed 'Herbier de M. Flobert, le cadet, 1778'. The title page reads 'Herbal or dried Garden, containing the usual plants, for both human and veterinary medicine, arranged according to the method of M. Tournefort, by M. Flobert, student at the Paris Veterinary School, May 11th MDCCLXXVIII.' On the same page there is a handwritten quotation from Linnaeus: 'For the botanist, a method is the thread of Ariadne; without its help, botany is mere chaos.' There follows a page of pen and wash images. They depict agricultural implements, veterinary instruments, and tools for shoeing animals, along with a quotation in French from Virgil's *Georgics*: 'Sans tous ces instruments, il n'est point de culture.' The floral specimens are labelled according to their French rather than their Latin names. In a traditionalist gesture, Nicolas uses the pre-Linnaean taxonomy devised by the late seventeenth-century French botanist Joseph Tournefort (1656–1708), director of the Paris *jardin du roi* in the early days when it was primarily intended for medicinal botany.[12]

In addition to its formal botanical content, the flora is respectfully and affectionately dedicated to the student's father, fondly remembered as the man who first taught his son the names of the plants. The inscribed dedication tactfully implies that this son has enjoyed an education far superior to that of his father. It also opens a small window onto an already distant intimate scene of instruction:

Though you have no knowledge of nature, you love it and it is the plant kingdom that you love above all. I know that you have endeavoured, as far as your condition has allowed, to acquire a knowledge of the plants proper to curing the maladies of animals. You even taught me the names and the uses of some of them at an age when the mind is scarce able to receive or to retain particular impressions.[13]

That dedication tells us that Nicolas was, in the language of the day, a man of feeling, a man who had enjoyed a generous and sympathetic relationship with his father. It was a good foundation for later ambitions and for relations with his own sons.

The third item from Alfort is the *brevet*. When Nicolas graduated from Alfort in October 1780, he was awarded his *brevet*. A nicely ambiguous word, *brevet* is best translated as 'patent', in the older sense of an open letter issued by a monarch to confer a privilege. The wording of the *brevet* enacts the potent legal fiction that the patent is granted by the individual action of the monarch from whom all wisdom and all authority derive. The text conveys the flavour of the professional world of the last decade of the Ancien Régime.

On this day, the King being at Versailles, His Majesty having deemed it fitting for the good of his service and for the benefit of the realm to order by the act of his Council that there shall be conferred Letters of Royal Privilege upon the Pupils of the Royal Schools of Veterinary Medicine, who have for four years pursued in the said Schools their course of study imparting the knowledge of livestock and of the diseases to which they are subject, and being well appraised of the religion, the competence and the experience of Nicolas FLOBERT who according to the testimony of the Professors of the said School has followed for four years the course of Study at the Paris Royal School of Veterinary Medicine, his Majesty has conferred upon him this present Patent to exercise the art of Veterinary Medicine, or treatment of the diseases of livestock in the Province and Generality of Paris and even beyond that said Province, if he be called there in the event of epidemic disease, after the treatment of which he will return into the said Province in which he has his establishment, without that for reason of his exercise of the said art he suffer interference at the hands of any individual, any craft, guild or other corporate body, and thus is it ordered by the said act of the Council of August 11th 1780. Signed Louis.[14]

This document is not the equivalent of a modern professional qualification. When we examine the operative terms in the text, several differences emerge. In addition to the powerful fiction of royal privilege, the brevet allows the holder to practice veterinary medicine exclusively in his province of origin, and elsewhere only in exceptional circumstances. France in 1780 was still a federation of provinces, each with its proud local peculiarities that the Revolution would struggle to erase, in the name of the Republic 'one and indivisible'.

IN THE SUMMER OF 1780, at the age of twenty-six, Nicolas Flaubert graduated and began work in the village of Bagneux, in the position recently vacated by his elder brother Jean-Baptiste, who now moved to Nogent. Nicolas was married in 1783 at the age of twenty-nine to a woman three years his junior, the daughter of a village master-surgeon. Among men of professional status, late marriage, preferably within the trade and to a younger woman, was a salient fact of late eighteenth-century demography.[15] Achille-Cléophas, the first of their two children, was born in the house where his mother was born, in the village of Maizières-la-Grande-Paroisse, twenty-five kilometres to the east of Nogent.

Within the year, in 1784, the new family made that day's journey to Nogent. The move may well have been prompted by the need to escape from hostile local gossip. Nicolas was at the centre of a minor financial scandal, which has left distinct traces in the regional archives. He came to the attention of the authorities after one or two of his clients complained that he was overcharging them for his services. The veterinary school archives at Alfort record the opinion that Nicolas is 'good at his work, but he runs up expenses, and presents bills for exorbitant amounts, a thing which obliges *Monsieur l'Intendant* only to employ him with some caution'. In May 1784 Nicolas was summoned to Troyes, the regional capital. There he received an official warning that 'if in future he were ever subject to similar complaints he would be severely punished'.[16] Henceforth, Nicolas would be aware that the all-powerful local *Intendant* was watching him. That cherished *Brevet de Privilégié du Roy* was a splendid thing, but it was evidently not a magic lantern.

Newly qualified, Nicolas was now working in the farms and villages all across his home province of Champagne. He was sent wherever needed, to tackle the effects of epidemic disease among valuable livestock. He worked in collaboration with local veterinarians, instructing them in effective forms of treatment. Here was the problem. He was a young man in a superior role, and it was all too easy to make enemies. In his mind, those high fees were his just reward. In the mind of a peevish and impecunious farmer, they were a piece of effrontery. There, in those daily farmyard encounters, was the whole drama of modernity. Nicolas was learning that the local heroes of enlightenment, with *brevet* in hand, might have to endure being forever an object of untutored suspicion. The Revolution, regarded as a boisterous Festival of Reason, would eventually add to the problem.

In June 1786, only two years after those first complaints, we find Nicolas's brother Jean-Baptiste complaining, in a letter to the Comte de Brienne, that *he* has been wrongly accused of presenting exorbitant bills, when the real culprit is his younger brother, Nicolas.

PROVINCIAL FAMILIES, long settled in a landscape intimately known, will cherish the names of the three or four villages that circumscribe a shared history. For the Flaubert brothers, dwelling on the threshold of modernity, their special villages were Bagneux, Anglure and Mazières-la-Grande-Paroisse. They are all within a day's journey of each other, and all favourably located along the network of fertile river valleys where the Aube meets the Seine. At the centre of this rural constellation was the town of Nogent-sur-Seine. This was where Achille-Cléophas spent the years of his boyhood, among the educated middling fraction of the provincial urban elite.

The everyday life of such a place was infinitely interesting to an intelligent child. In a busy market town, with a population of around three thousand, there was plenty to see: wide green meadows, a deep river with an array of bridges, watermills and lock gates, as well as ships coming and going. Sitting in the middle of 'vast and superb prairielands', Nogent gathered both grain and hay for shipment downriver to Paris. The grain trade linked the town to the swift ebb and flow of the market. There was a regular riverboat service to Paris and a considerable fleet of shipping. Within the complex political framework of the Ancien Régime, Nogent was among those central regions more profoundly penetrated by capitalism, with improved communications and greater administrative centralisation.

The town enjoyed a splendid situation: 'well-built, neat, and airy', at the point where the Seine became navigable. There were 'beautiful walks on the banks of the Seine, which command a fine prospect of the country and of the navigation'.[17] Goods on their way to Paris passed through the town, to the sound of heavy wagons rumbling along the main street. The long-distance coach-service, the diligence, called at the inn on the town square. Sailors disembarked from the riverboats and headed for the brothels near the quayside. At the centre of things, between the canal and the river, there stood a narrow island with two fine stone bridges recently built, the pride of the town. The road to Paris ran downhill, straight across the meadows, through lines of poplar trees. In winter the meadows were half-flooded from the waters of the Seine, and in summer the cornfields were decorated with poppies.[18]

Beyond a handful of picturesque external details, we know very little about Achille-Cléophas's riverside childhood years in Nogent. Evidently his attachment to the place was strong and silent. We do know that the older man returned repeatedly, in the summer with his young family, to the town that had been the scene of his boyhood. Eventually, he bought four acres of land near the river, in one of the spots where he used to play. Nogent would be the place where the heroic story had begun, the place of enduring love in a life beset by perilous uncertainty. It is thus slightly puzzling that the archive has preserved no distinct memories of this early life. On the subject of Nogent, the recollections recorded by his junior colleagues are surprisingly meagre. Was it perhaps his intention to draw a veil of silence over something disagreeable?

The explanation for this reticence may well lie in the exceptionally painful circumstances surrounding the death of Achille-Cléophas's father, Nicolas Flaubert, in 1814. In violation of strict chronology, the story of that death can conveniently be told at this point. In February 1814, with the French nation in a state of exhausted misery, with Napoleon and his armies in disarray, the town of Nogent was besieged for two days by invading Russian troops. They came in from the east, en route for Paris. In a quixotically defiant gesture, Nogent resisted their advance, and this resistance was met with an artillery bombardment. This destroyed one of the town's stone bridges and set fire to several buildings. As the fire took hold and began to spread, families who had been hiding in the cellars of their houses fled the town. Some fifty dwellings were burnt to the ground and many of the rest were looted.

The victorious Russian soldiers entered the town and took a gleeful revenge for the recent sufferings of their own country at the hands of the French. Typically, rationally, the predators seized food and money and any other portable property; their less fortunate victims were subject to wanton destruction, insults, violence, rape.[19] Atrocity stories from Nogent duly appeared in the French press. Amongst their other deeds, Russian soldiers were said to have cut off the finger of an old woman in order to steal her ring.[20] At times such as these, there will be a spike in the death-rate. Nicolas Flaubert, survivor of revolutions, resident of Nogent, died in the first week of May 1814, at the age of fifty-seven. In view of the characteristic longevity of his genetic line, this was an early death.

Achille-Cléophas was twenty-nine at this point and on the threshold of professional success. We do not know what Achille-Cléophas knew or believed about his father's death. On the other hand, we do know that the ruins of some of the buildings destroyed in the siege of 1814 were still standing in the early 1830s when Achille-Cléophas and his young family came to Nogent for the summer.[21] Any moderately curious child would want to know the story of those incongruous ruins. But it would not be unusual, in that generation, for the details of such events to be tacitly deleted from the collective memory.

BE THAT AS IT MAY, in various letters from Nogent, written in later years, we may catch a glimpse of the distinctive pleasures of the place. Family letters mention the distinctively slow sing-song intonations of local speech,[22] the marvellous fishing expeditions, the long walks through the countryside and up into the hills.[23] Summer journeys from Rouen to Nogent were a feature of family life in the 1830s: 'the vineyards […] and the white houses, the long dusty road, and the line of cropped elm-trees'.[24] This, the Nogent of later years, the place of summer holidays with cousins, is celebrated in Gustave Flaubert's novel *Sentimental Education*. The novel is set in the 1840s, and the hero re-enacts closely the geographical pattern of Achille-Cléophas life, moving from village to town to city. From Nogent to Sens, from Sens to Paris.

The only account of Achille-Cléophas's childhood is to be found in the post-mortem biography of 1847. It offers no concrete details. 'From his early youth', says his perfectly deferential biographer, 'he was remarkable for his energy, which gave him an obvious superiority over his young companions, both in bodily exercises and in those of the mind. Thus, both at play and in his school work, he was consistently ahead of everyone else.'[25]

One can easily imagine a contrary response to this precocious excellence. It might read as follows. Even as a child, Achille-Cléophas was possessed by a fiercely competitive spirit. Whether he was playing with the other boys down by the river, or learning his letters from some indolent priest, he simply excelled. He always had to be the best. Everyone agreed that Achille-Cléophas was a boy who might go far. This country town was far too modest an arena for energy and talent such as his. Those of a more critical disposition, his peers or his siblings, might have added, under their breath, that such damned superiority would one day be sure to *end miserably*.

The complex truth of Achille-Cléophas's early life must lie somewhere in between these two accounts, the formally deferential and the intimately hostile. All the later evidence, from those who knew him, both family and colleagues, suggests a man of fiercely satirical rectitude, though they also agree that this formidable aggression was tempered or held in check by an essential benevolence. His patients adored him for his gentleness and his everyday compassion. But he was *opinionâtre*. Amongst other things, that means relentless. 'Opinionâtre en toutes choses', said one of his professional contemporaries.[26] He was diligent, tenacious, and persistent. But he was also stubborn, inflexible and unyielding. It is perfectly familiar now, this melancholy relentlessness, this sombre passion of men devoured by their work. In the 1790s, when Achille-Cléophas began to discover the wider world beyond his immediate family, it was still regarded as a potentially sinister psychological novelty. In the summer of 1789, all such questions were still far away in the future. For Achille-Cléophas the timeless and self-delighting flow of early childhood experience was about to be disturbed by events that would be infinitely perplexing. Within a few years, the everyday certainties of small-town family life would all be swept away.

Nogent, Sens, Paris, Rouen: these four place-names circumscribe the life of Achille-Cléophas. Three of these places are on the Seine, and the fourth, Sens, is on a tributary of the Seine. In a slightly fanciful psycho-geography, Achille-Cléophas is moving slowly downstream towards the sea. In later life, in the 1830s when he lived and worked in Rouen, he and his family regularly travelled back to the source, to Nogent, to the house of his boyhood on the rue de L'Etape de vin. You may get out, get on and get rich, but you return to your home town, Nogent-sur-Seine, ever loyal to the place you remember best.

This Nogent connection, on his father's side, was equally important to Gustave Flaubert. It gave him a substantial collection of country cousins along with a lone survivor of the older generation, his paternal grandmother, Marie-Apollonie Flaubert. She figures pleasantly in his early history as the distant source of regular New Year parcels packed with good things to eat. Marie-Apollonie died in 1832 when Gustave was ten, thus breaking his last intimate family link with the eighteenth century.

2

Fresh Corpses

The storms of Revolution, stirred up corresponding tempests in the passions of men, and overwhelmed not a few in a total ruin of their distinguished birthright as rational beings.

— PHILIPPE PINEL, *A Treatise on Insanity* (1806)

ON 17 APRIL 1792, at first light, a group of surprisingly important people has assembled in the dissection room at Le Bicêtre, the all-purpose hospital-prison-asylum complex just south of the city walls of Paris. The party includes two eminent philosopher-physicians, Cabanis and Pinel, along with a group of deputies from the National Assembly. They have gathered to witness a most interesting experiment. The prototype of a new device is about tested.

For the process to be swift and painless, it has been calculated that the heavy steel blade should drop from a height of fourteen feet. This is Enlightenment applied to the practicalities of execution. Three fresh cadavers have been supplied by the prison administration. Sanson, the executioner, lays the first cadaver face down and then releases the catch. The great blade falls, separating the head from the body. It works 'in a flash' said Cabanis, offering his congratulations to the makers of the ingenious contraption. At this point, according to popular memory, the executioner is heard to observe sadly, 'Splendid invention! As long as they don't get carried away with it [...]'. According to the same story, Prisoner A says to Prisoner B, 'That's what they mean by Equality. Everyone dies in the same way.' 'Yes indeed', says Prisoner B, 'what a leveller!'[1] Eight days later, the first public execution by guillotine takes place on the Place de Grève.

The first live subject is Jacques Pelletier, a convicted thief. The inventor of this 'instrument of separation', Dr Guillotin, will himself be guillotined at Le Bicêtre only a year later.[2]

IN LATE JANUARY 1793, the year in which the Revolution begins to devour its own, a man in his late thirties is standing near the fire in a village tavern, reading *Le Moniteur*. He shakes his head and frowns. He reads the news aloud to the company, trusting that they will share his anguish and his grief: Louis XVI was executed, two days ago. The patriot sitting in the corner has been listening. He sees an opportunity. Next day, Citizen Nicolas Flaubert is denounced to the local Revolutionary Committee as a royalist. Royalists are the enemy within. They have him arrested.

Defiant and apprehensive, he stands before his accusers. What possesses them? These men are his neighbours. He has known them for years. They are fired up with an impulsive mix of private envy and competitive patriotic enthusiasm. *Citizen* Flaubert! With sardonic emphasis on that new egalitarian prefix, he will now be *transported* – their gleeful, knowing euphemism – to Paris, two days down river. There he will face the Revolutionary Court, then the guillotine or if not the guillotine, then deportation to some tropical hellhole. The quick death or the slow death, it scarcely deserves to be called a choice.

Enter, at the last moment, a boy of seven. He is bright and self-assured, the eldest son of the accused. Well-tutored by his mother, he pleads for his father's life with such precocious eloquence, such transparent purity of heart. Nicolas Flaubert's accusers are moved. They confer. They relent. One of the committee, perhaps the lawyer, wins them over. He has read Rousseau. He is educated, politically ambitious, but also a man of feeling. The rest, made of plainer stuff, realise that Nicolas Flaubert is an excellent vet, whatever else he is. The village needs him, to keep the horses working. Enjoying their own largesse, they tell him to watch his tongue in future.

In the other version of the same story, Nicolas Flaubert owes his survival to a fortunate accident. He has been condemned to death and on the morning of the execution the cart taking him to the scaffold breaks down, a short distance from the prison. The condemned men are taken back to the prison; the next day is XX Thermidor. The prisoner walks free.[3]

REAL OR IMAGINED, or poised creatively between the two, these stories were cherished items of Flaubert family legend. This was their memory of the Revolution, their lesson in the perils of political enthusiasm, a story to pass on to your son on his sixteenth birthday and a healing image at a time when memories of Revolutionary violence were being erased from the public sphere.[4] Seventy years after the event, it made such a good after-dinner story that Edmond Goncourt thought it worth writing down.

With such events, whatever their reality, there is no simple recall of the facts. There is a shared experience, an array of evolving memories. In this enclosed, collective, trans-generational narrative process there is only a shadowy distinction between the imagined and the real. It follows that to correct the family story from the historical record is perhaps to overlook the intimate purpose of that story.[5]

I propose to take that story seriously, as a fiction, as a collective psychological artefact. Considered as a miniature political romance, it brings together all the best Oedipal ingredients: the death of a king, the death threatened to the man who wept so incontinently, the death averted by the precocious eloquence of a mere child. The more contingent details – the time and the place of the telling of the story – are also part of the meaning. Gustave Flaubert told the story one evening in late January 1863. The date catches the eye. That was seventy years, almost to the day, since the execution of Louis XVI. (Significantly, the Goncourts had published two books about the Revolution, back in 1854 and 1855.)

Prompted by the impending anniversary, perhaps the after-dinner conversation had turned spontaneously to the strange days of January 1793. That date was also significant in another way. Flaubert's father, Achille-Cléophas, the child in the story, died on 15 January 1846. Flaubert was thus telling this story in the week of the eighteenth anniversary of his father's death. This story, told at this moment, encapsulates a range of reactions to the death of a father. The father, Nicolas, weeps for the death of his king. The son, Achille-Cléophas, speaks words from the mother and prevents a death. The grandson, Gustave, remembering a death witnessed, tells a story of a death evaded.

All in all, the Goncourt story is a richly tendentious improvisation on the paternal theme. It stages an inversion of the customary and decorous transmission of identity and social status from father to son. In this instance, the son, while still a young boy, acts to ensure the survival of his father. Telling the story when he does and as he does, Gustave Flaubert is placing himself in a magically unbroken line that reaches back to his paternal grandfather.

That line was almost broken. Hidden away in the folds of this after-dinner story is the fact that three of Gustave's four grandparents died before he was born. Three out of four is more than enough for one family, though scarcely unusual for those heroic, high-mortality decades of Revolution and Empire. As already described, his paternal grandfather, Nicolas Flaubert, died in May 1814, victim of the social chaos attending the fall of the First Empire. His maternal grandmother, Charlotte-Justine, died in 1793, a few days after giving birth. His maternal grandfather, Jean-Baptiste, died in 1803, in his early thirties.

His paternal grandmother, Marie-Apolline, was the only survivor. She lived on to the age of seventy-seven and she was the recipient, in her last years, of dutiful New Year letters from her schoolboy grandson Gustave. She died in 1832, leaving the boy a large piece of flower-print silk, cut from one of her ball gowns. We know of this object because, twelve years later, in September 1846, Gustave mentions using it as a special cloth to decorate the improvised shrine where the copious love-letters from his new mistress, Louise Colet, were hidden away from the gaze of his recently widowed mother. The shrine in question was set up inside the writing desk which had belonged to Gustave's beloved younger sister, Caroline, who had died from complications in childbirth earlier in the same year.[6]

Like the story told to the Goncourts, Gustave's shrine is a richly symbolic arrangement of cherished objects. The conjunction of the piece of silk, the writing desk and the letters, creates a connection between the four women in his life, one living, one widowed, and two dead: Flaubert's lover, his mother, his paternal grandmother and his sister. The shrine speaks of an alternative family history, a genealogical fable in which desire is transmitted down a circuitous female line, avoiding his widowed mother, and reaching back to the now distant days of his grandmother's ball-gown-wearing Ancien Régime girlhood.

Finally, it is worth imagining the consequences had Gustave's imprudent, and supposedly royalist grandfather been deported or executed for his alleged political opinions. The life of his grandson Gustave would have been different. Consider a plausible possible history. The widowed Marie-Apolline Flaubert of 1794 sinks into poverty. Her clever younger son, Achille-Cléophas, is not sent away in 1796 to the College de Sens for an expensive education. He does not scale the ladder of the medical profession. His (second) son, Gustave, is not born in 1821 in a big house to a rich father with an illustrious name. Without that material foundation of assured leisure created by the father, the insidiously exquisite, labour-intensive prose of *Madame Bovary* will not be written.

WORKING FROM THE HISTORICAL RECORD, we can augment and rectify that family oral tradition in some detail. The story proper began in September 1792 when Nicolas Flaubert was commissioned to work with those peasants who now found themselves responsible for livestock that had been the property of the previous government. This livestock was now to be regarded as a national asset.[7] The fact that Nicolas had previously been in trouble for overcharging was now no obstacle to his advancement. The war was going very badly. Since the summer of 1792, Prussian forces had been pushing over the frontiers in the north east of France.

The political authority of the beleaguered infant Republic now began to reach ever deeper into the everyday life of the population. *La patrie en danger*: the nation was under attack, from without and from within. There was no neutral ground. In March 1793 it was decreed that every commune must establish a watch committee, responsible for 'searching out political offenders, checking passports, cross-examining strangers and requisitioning for arms.'[8] By July 1793, Nicolas Flaubert was fully enrolled in the war effort, commissioned as a military transport contractor, 'in the name of the French Republic, one and indivisible'.

The text of his commission is of some interest. As well as describing the details of his physical appearance, the document testifies to those more elusive qualities of political orthodoxy and civic virtue. It reads as follows:

> In view of the favourable reports we have received concerning the patriotism, the good conduct and the competence of citizen Nicolas Flaubert […] aged thirty-six, five feet three inches tall, brown hair and eyebrows, blue eyes, ordinary forehead, round face, round chin – we have appointed him to the position of *maréchal des logis* [cavalry sergeant] in the crew in charge of the transport of military food supplies [presumably grain] […] with a salary of ninety livres per month, to run from 15 July 1793 – on condition that the aforesaid citizen carry out all instructions that will be issued to him in the interests of the service, that he devote himself to the interests of the

service as if they were his own, that he provide himself with a horse and a
uniform in accordance with the regulations adopted by the Company and
of which he has been informed.[9]

This was a natural step for a man in his position. It enabled him to avoid
conscription, even though it exposed him to financial temptation and
to neighbourly envy, insidious powers that would soon prove almost as
destructive as any of those that one might encounter on the battlefield.

A few weeks later, on 23 August 1793, mass mobilisation was declared.

> Henceforth, until our enemies have been driven from the territory of the
> Republic, all the French are in permanent requisition for army service. The
> young men shall go to battle; the married men shall forge arms and trans-
> port provisions; the women shall make tents and clothes, and shall serve in
> hospitals; the children shall turn old linen into lint; the old men shall repair
> to the public places, to stimulate the courage of the warriors and preach the
> unity of the Republic and the hatred of kings.[10]

In September 1793, for fear of the enemy within, the Convention passed
the Law of Suspects. Under this law, committees with powers of arrest
were to be established in every commune. The death penalty would be
imposed on anyone who 'either by their conduct, their contacts, their
words or their writings, showed themselves to be supporters of tyranny,
of federalism, or to be enemies of liberty'. 'Suspect' was defined in such
vague terms that it positively encouraged the practice of denunciation.[11]
The enemies of liberty could be the people next door. Whatever else it
achieved, the new law was an incitement to neighbourly malice, especially
in the towns. It has been estimated that around one million individuals
were imprisoned or brought under surveillance because of their political
views in 1793–4, 'roughly the same number as fought in the war'.[12] Nicolas
Flaubert was about to be one of that unfortunate million.

Within weeks of beginning work as a military transport contractor, Nicolas Flaubert was in trouble. In September, the month just after
the harvest, the time when large quantities of grain are on the move, he
was denounced by the General Council in Nogent. He was arrested, and
imprisoned and seals were placed upon his property, pending investigation. With the help of a sympathetic moderate deputy, Nicolas's wife
Marie-Apolline now organised a campaign for his release. From all across

the locality, from the villages where Nicolas Flaubert had worked with the animals, petitions were sent to the National Convention. Their message was simple. The man is indispensable. Our horses will die without his expert care.

The petitions had their effect. Early in January 1794, Nicolas Flaubert was provisionally released from prison. Within two weeks though, he was arrested once again. He evidently had powerful enemies on the local revolutionary committee. The mood of the hour was exceptionally volatile. It was only a year since the killing of the king. In the southern city of Toulon, recently recaptured from the English, the anniversary of the execution of Louis XVI was being celebrated by having wax figures representing the kings of Europe decapitated in public. Belligerent patriotic emotion allowed for no moral ambiguity. Public expressions of doubt or dissent, *propos inciviques*, were a criminal offence.

In Paris, on 14 January, a letter was delivered to the National Convention denouncing Nicolas Flaubert and his business partner for fraud in their military transport enterprise. On the next day *Le Moniteur*, official journal of record, carried the following brief item: 'The National Convention decrees that Claude Moreau, military transport contractor, and Flobert, veterinary artist from Nogent-sur-Seine, with the rank of sergeant in one of Moreau's workgroups, will be brought before the Revolutionary Court there to be judged according to the laws.'[13]

Flaubert's employer, Claude Moreau, was sentenced to death. In *Le Moniteur* for 4 March 1794, we read the following announcement:

> Claude Moreau, aged thirty-five years, born in Tonerre, department of the Yonne, contractor for military transport and food supplies, formerly wagon-master, convicted of fraud in the supply of horses for the Republic, has been condemned to death. Nicolas Flobert, aged thirty-six years, born in Saint-Just, near Sezanne, resident in Nogent-sur-Seine, convicted of having voiced unpatriotic [*inciviques*] and counter-revolutionary opinions, has been condemned to deportation.[14]

Nicolas defended himself resourcefully, and he was acquitted on the charge of fraud. He was about to be released when he was denounced, once again. This time he was accused of *propos inciviques et contre-revolutionnaires*.[15] On close inspection, Nicolas had been accused of two legally distinct offences. Counter-revolutionary utterance was the more

serious of the two. This included 'speaking against conscription or pro-
posing the restoration of the monarchy, the dissolution of the National
Convention or disparagement of constituted authorities, even those of
one's village' and attracted the death penalty.[16] The dissident utterance,
the *propos incivique*, was less serious. It attracted the lesser sentence of
deportation, typically a lingering tropical death.[17] The archives of the
Revolutionary Court document the fact that Nicolas was acquitted of the
charge of counter-revolutionary utterances. He was found guilty of the
lesser offence and sentenced accordingly to deportation.[18]

At this point, early in March 1794, Nicolas wrote to his ally, the deputy,
setting out his case:

> I was acquitted and declared innocent, unanimously, of this of offence [of
> fraud]. I was about to be set free when my accuser, who had vowed to destroy
> me, desperate when he saw the zeal with which more than eighty communes
> supported me, accused me of uttering certain *propos inciviques*. A thing
> incredible and unheard of! On the strength of this vague and false depo-
> sition, I have been condemned to deportation, on 9 ventôse [27 February
> 1794]. Among the eighty communes who need my services and who have all
> suffered great losses since my imprisonment, forty-five had expressly given
> me certificates of citizenship and good conduct.
>
> I shall not at this point go into detail of the many successful cures which
> I have effected in the six leagues around the town of Troyes in the area where
> I live. The evidence is there in the many petitions and testimonials drawn
> up in my favour by nearly one hundred communes who are desperate for
> my release.[19]

Whatever one's offence, this was not a good moment to fall into the hands
of the Republic's hastily improvised judicial system, though due process
was more likely to be observed by the courts in Paris than in the provinces, where political justice was often dispensed by 'outsiders operating
under the eye of *représentants en mission* seeking a reputation for zeal'.[20]
At the height of the Terror, then, Nicolas Flaubert spent eight months in
Le Bicêtre, the main prison outside Paris, pending an appeal against his
sentence of deportation.

To put that another way, Achille-Cléophas spent those same eight
months, at the age of nine, fearing, believing, denying and remembering
that he might never see his father again. I picture the boy repeating in

his mind the whole recent sequence of real and imagined events. It was an infernal sequence of nine commonplace verbs: denounced, arrested, charged, acquitted, denounced, imprisoned, condemned, deported and then vanished. Such prolonged and corrosive uncertainty, experienced at this age, might leave its insidiously toxic residue of despair.

SITUATED OUT AT GENTILLY, three miles from the centre of Paris, in the southern suburbs, Le Bicêtre was a voracious piece of national-moral machinery, perfectly engineered for the ancient task of the polis, to discipline and punish. Indifferently functioning as hospital, prison and asylum, Le Bicêtre lived in the popular imagination as an imposing neo-classical receptacle of all the miseries. This was the place you disappeared into, the day your luck ran out. Chronically damp and overcrowded, in the summer of 1794 Le Bicêtre housed prisoners condemned to death as well as those awaiting deportation.

In the early 1790s, the prison yard at Le Bicêtre saw the opening scene of one of the more spectacular rituals of punishment. Every month, groups of convicts from the cities of the north arrived, awaiting deportation. Then, twice a year, in May and September, in the main yard, *la chaîne* formed up: long lines of men chained together, ready for the journey to the coast and subsequent deportation. Even if you had never seen it, there was a good chance that, in the year 1794, you could imagine finding yourself *in it*.

La chaîne was perhaps the most insidiously compelling image of the hour. It had a distinct cultural currency: Louis-Léopold Boilly, the contemporary painter of modern life, depicted it soberly in 1792; Victor Hugo dramatised it in his Gothic tale *The Last Day of a Condemned Man* in 1830; a civil servant described it meticulously in 1890, this time from archival evidence, as something disgraceful from the bad old days, now happily abolished. The following scene draws upon that archival evidence. This is the scene that Achille-Cléophas could have pictured to himself, repeatedly, at any point in the next fifty years of his life. Imagined or remembered, it was what was once about to happen to his father.

On the day, the number of prison-guards was doubled. Heavy carts, followed by soldiers, arrive in the yard. The carts carry big wooden chests containing an assortment of chains and iron collars and grey canvas garments. Awakened by the unusual noise, prisoners appear at the windows of their cells. They curse, they cheer, and they mock. Prisoners listed for deportation are brought down into the yard, twenty-six at a time. They are ordered to strip off. Doctors, elegant and disdainful in their white cravats and their black frock coats, examine the prisoners. All the usual tales of incapacity are treated with cold professional scepticism. The doctors certify them all *bons pour le bagne* (fit for deportation).

The prisoners are each given their grey canvas uniforms, *the taffeta*, in prison slang. The great wooden chests are opened. Out come the long heavy chains, *the strings*. Prisoners are brought forward in pairs. Tight-fitting triangular iron collars with hinges are positioned around each man's neck. There is a different size collar for each different size of head. These are *the tassels*. Each man kneels at a little portable anvil and a blacksmith with a great iron hammer crushes the hinge on the collar. The thing is now impossible to open. To avoid injury, the prisoner must keep absolutely still, as he lays his neck upon the anvil. At this point it is good form to curse and swear, making as much noise as possible. The very boldest will affect an air of cynical bravado. This perplexes the curious, moralising, educated observer. Anyone seen weeping, his fellows will mock relentlessly. The collared man is then attached by a small chain to the main chain, *the string*. The string slowly acquires its full complement, thirteen pairs of *tassels*, all in *taffeta*. As a finishing touch, a trusty with a long pair of scissors cuts off everyone's hair and whiskers.

Straw is spread across the yard. The prisoners will spend the night there, restlessly awake in their unfamiliar collars and chains. At first light, next day, the special transportation carts arrive. The cart is a curious thing, merely a long horizontal iron beam with wheels at each end. The string of prisoners sits on the beam, back to back, in pairs, their collars chained to the beam. Then away they go: exemplary turpitude, cropped and shackled. From here, humiliated, defiant or desolate, they make their way into the west, through towns and villages, an instructive spectacle, heading for the penal establishments on the Atlantic coast, Brest, L'Orient and Rochefort.[21]

A simple question arises. Why was Nicolas Flaubert not simply deported in the national chain that left Le Bicêtre at the beginning of May 1794? Perhaps the process of deportation was temporarily suspended, either because of the allied naval blockade, or because of the military crisis in the western provinces. We find a possible explanation in the records of the Alfort veterinary school. On 25 October 1794, while Nicolas was still in prison, Alfort issued a duplicate copy of his original veterinary qualification. This document must have played a part in his wife's continuing campaign for his acquittal. That campaign was certainly not helped by the actions of his wife's sister, Helene Marchand. She was arrested in September 1794, 'accused of fanaticism and religious propaganda […] preaching on street corners, roaming the streets and crossroads singing hymns'.[22]

Achille-Cléophas surely visited his father at some point during the long months of his imprisonment. There were regular passenger boats up and down the Seine, between Nogent and Paris, and then Le Bicêtre was only a few miles from the city centre. According to the prison archives, the visiting room was set up to prevent physical contact between the prisoners and their visitors. Visitors were confined to a narrow corridor with a double row of heavy bars between them and the inmates.

There was father, wearing the ugly prison uniform, the heavy canvas trousers and the smock, half black and half grey. He doesn't know it yet, but his brown hair has started to turn grey. He makes linen, or metal buttons, twelve hours a day. The first few days are the worst, he says. You sit in your cell, feeling sorry for yourself, then angry, then sad, then angry again. You weep and curse, all at the same time. Then you hear the sound of cheerful conversation next door. You get a grip, you settle down to work. There is money to be made, little luxuries to be bought.[23]

Meanwhile Marie-Apolline, his wife, was organising a second appeal on his behalf. By mid-summer, events on the national political stage were slowly turning in her favour. The arrest and execution of Robespierre and his friends in July 1794, sparked rumours that everyone imprisoned under the Law of Suspects would be freed immediately. Conmen selling bogus releases did a good trade. Excited crowds gathered at prisons gates. Deputies were besieged by the friends and relatives of prisoners, petitioning for their release. In Marseilles, the crowd broke into the prison. In Paris, the Convention began to undo the laws that had made possible 'the system of the Terror'. In October, the marquis de Sade walked free, on account of his many patriotic works. Deputies began to worry that genuine counter-revolutionaries might be released.[24]

In December 1794, after months of recruiting influential acquaintances to lend their support to the cause, Marie-Apolline Flaubert appeared in person before the National Convention in Paris. There she delivered an appeal on behalf of her imprisoned husband. She speaks the obligatory, impassioned, heroic language of the hour:

Representatives of the People, Fathers of the Nation,
Justice and humanity are the order of the day: you yourselves have made it
so; this news resounds across all of France; and it encourages me to appear in
person in order to claim a benefit common to all the French. I am an unfortunate wife; my beloved children have been orphans for the last seventeen
months, ever since the detention of their father who has now spent eight
months in the dreadful cells of the Bicêtre prison. My unfortunate husband,
Nicolas Flaubert, was condemned to be deported by the Revolutionary Court,
in those days of fear, when Robespierre and his agents, believing themselves
to be above the law, acted in contempt of law and humanity; he is not accused
or convicted under any law. Legislators, I ask of you only that his case be
put before the Committee of General Security. Fortified by all the evidence
of his innocence, I hope with a modest confidence that this concession will
bring about the restitution of the liberty to which I lay claim.[25]

Her request was forwarded to the Committee of Public Safety. On 23
January 1795, her husband was acquitted and released from prison.

RELEASED FROM PRISON, but not from the memory. Within a few
years there would be much debate upon the public health effects of the
Revolution. Among those who had suffered under the Terror, there
were several obvious and immediate physical symptoms. Hair turned
white, eyebrows fell out, faces wrinkled and eyes became infected. Under
Robespierre, there were more aneurisms than usual; and midwives
reported many more difficult deliveries, as if babies were reluctant to
emerge into a wicked world.

There were also more elusive psychological effects. People went deaf,
or lost their memory.[26] Such oblivion might well be a blessing in disguise.
The Revolution could otherwise possess the imagination entirely, causing
the departure of 'the real and respectable man.' Philippe Pinel, the French
physician who pioneered the humane 'moral treatment' of the insane,
describes once such case. He was 'the man who lost his head'. His tragicomic story rivals the most fervid inventions of the Gothic. It lingers in
the imagination as an epitome of the 1790s.

A celebrated watchmaker, at Paris [...] was infatuated with the chimera of perpetual motion, and to effect this discovery, he set to work with indefatigable

ardour. From unremitting attention to the object of his enthusiasm, coinciding with the influence of revolutionary disturbance, his imagination was greatly heated, his sleep was interrupted, and, at length, a complete derangement of the understanding took place. His case was marked by a most whimsical illusion of the imagination. He fancied that he had lost his head on the scaffold; that it had been thrown promiscuously among the heads of many other victim; that the judges, heaving repented of their cruel sentence, had ordered those heads to be restored to their respective owners, and placed upon their respective shoulders; but that, in consequence of an unfortunate mistake, the gentlemen, who had the management of that business, had placed upon his shoulders the head of one of his unhappy companions. The idea of this whimsical exchange of his head, occupied his thoughts night and day; […] Nothing could equal the extravagant overflowings of his heated brain. 'Look at these teeth,' he constantly cried; 'Mine were exceedingly handsome; – these are rotten and decayed.'[27]

3

A Radical Education

Will you forgive me, gentlemen, this digression that has slipped out in spite
of myself? I thought I would offer only a brief reminiscence; but where is
the man who, in speaking of the ills he has suffered, is able to set any proper
limit to his thoughts? Suffering seems to bestow the right to say everything;
the heart overflows unawares, and just when one seems to have forgotten
everything the incontinent heart takes its revenge.

— MARC-ANTOINE PETIT, *The Influence of the French Revolution on
Public Health* (1806)

L IKE A MAN RETURNING FROM THE DEAD, Nicolas Flaubert made
his way home. Having survived the Terror, he would hope to dis-
appear back into his family circle, safe from the hostile gaze of
the authorities. As a consequence of his seventeen months in prison, his
family was now short of money. They would, nevertheless, send their
oldest boy to the very best school. Education was a good investment.
All the exclusive old careers were opening up. Qualifications were going
to be the new currency. The boy was obviously clever. He could become
anything: a lawyer or even a doctor. They resolved to make all the necessary sacrifices. 'Though there was little to spare, the family saved up
what they could.'[1]

Thus it was that in the autumn of the year 1795, a few weeks before
his eleventh birthday, this talented child was transported the thirty-odd
miles from the scene of his boyhood to the neighbouring town of Sens. It
was a slow and fatiguing day's journey, but his brilliant career was about
to begin, so they said.

Achille-Cléophas was educated, for the next seven years, from 1795 until 1802, as *pensionnaire*, a boarding pupil, at the Collège de Sens. To be there, in that school, in that town, in those years after Thermidor: the experience was going to be disconcertingly instructive, in ways that were not documented in the school prospectus. The college itself had recently been housed, after some initial improvisation, on a new site in the old convent, a national asset recently confiscated from the Catholic church. The college buildings formed a portion of the old city walls, and this picturesque position, looking out, at the edge of the city, offered to all the students an amusing vision of alternative worlds. In one direction, you could look out within the walls, along the narrow echoing streets of the old city. In the other direction, you could look out, beyond the walls, to the grove of trees and the open countryside beyond.[2]

Somewhere, far away to the northwest, at the end of a white dusty road, there lay the great city of Paris. Any ambitious new boy, proud of his progress in mathematics, gazing out towards that imagined destination, might calculate the duration of the hundred-mile horse-and-cart journey to the capital. The riverboat service would be much quicker, though much more expensive. The important question was when? Woven into all the adult talk of war, there was contentious talk of equality. As a citizen of the Republic, you knew only that your future was likely to be different from everything that had gone before.

FROM THE EVIDENCE OF THE LOCAL ARCHIVES, Sens welcomed the Revolution with exceptional enthusiasm. The municipal government was Jacobin for most of the time from July 1794 until November 1799.[3] Sens possessed all the material ingredients for a volatile political culture: a navigable river and a national highway, to link with events in Paris; encircling city walls and narrow streets, to contain and channel an excited crowd; spacious public squares, suitable for large impromptu meetings; a multitude of old churches where political clubs could gather and conspire against each other. Add to all of these distinctive local features a contentiously literate and mutually hostile elite of lawyers, doctors, clerics and merchants, their political opinions nourished and inflamed by the pamphlets and newspapers that issued from competing local print shops. With a population of around ten thousand and a long history as a centre of ecclesiastical administration, Sens was a place where ideas readily acquired a certain material force.

The last five years had been tumultuous. The city had been stripped of many of its ancient privileges. It had lost its archbishop, its law courts, its college and its two seminaries.[4] In the space of a few months, the ritual, the personnel and all the poetic paraphernalia of centuries of faith had been terminated. In November 1790, there had been the first auctions of confiscated church property and then the new oath of allegiance to the Civil Constitution of Clergy. It was all infinitely divisive. How were the people to catch up with their leaders? If you were a friend of the Revolution you must obviously be an enemy of the church. In the autumn of 1795, when Achille-Cléophas arrived in Sens, the campaign against the embedded powers of superstition and fanaticism, also known as the Catholic church, was not yet over.

De-Christianisation was a new word, portentously new. For the citizens of Sens in the autumn of 1795, the word already had a history. In November 1790 the local cathedral canons had assembled in the Chapel of Perseverance to hear that the cathedral chapter was legally dissolved.[5] In the summer of 1792, the boisterous ragged army of the Revolution, the *fédérés*, had marched through Sens on their way from Marseille to Paris, raising a great cloud of dust and singing the fiery new anthem of the Republic, the *Marseillaise*. In January 1793, the Carmelite nuns had been evicted and their convent sold off. Taken in by local families, the nuns set up a little school, with pictures of the saints on the walls. Frowned upon, for being 'attached to ancient prejudices and superstitious practices', the school was eventually forced to close.[6] Later in 1793, the college was closed down and its substantial assets in property, worth 30,000 livres per year, were sold off. The main building was then converted to a salt-petre works and a prison for captured Austrian soldiers.[7] Education in the town came to a halt.

There was more to come. In November 1793, the revolutionary army from Lyon passed through Sens. With the support of local patriots from the clubs, the soldiers chopped down crosses, and built bonfires of religious images and relics.[8] The Cathedral of St Stephen was efficiently stripped of the company of stone saints that had adorned its west front since the twelfth century. Only St Stephen himself, holding the book of the law in his hand, escaped the gleeful hammer of popular iconoclasm.[9] The Place de la Cathédrale was renamed Place de la Liberté.[10]

By the late spring of 1794, across the nation, Catholic worship had come to a halt: 'most churches were closed, nearly all priests had abdicated, been imprisoned, gone into hiding, married or fled'.[11] In November of that year, to consolidate the still-fragile cultural revolution, a decree banished all religious instruction from schools. Fanaticism and superstition were to be replaced by moral education and civic training.[12] Pupils were to be given copies of the officially approved Republican catechism, a pocket-sized book with a virtuous and patriotic thought for every day of the year, indispensable for the children of liberty.[13] Great rhetorical violence was deemed necessary to undo the ancestral–monarchical–clerical loyalties of the population. The motto on the title page of one such publication sets the tone: 'Hell spews forth Kings. Reason destroys them.'[14]

There were, of course, odd twists and turns in the local history of the Revolution. Church and state had been formally separated in February 1795. Paradoxically, at that point, there was a revival in Catholic worship. Inevitably, along with the restoration of the signs and symbols of Christianity, there arose in the minds of the faithful, a certain stubborn and surreptitious counter-revolutionary humour. Church bells rang out once again. Refractory priests urged the restoration of the monarchy. The forbidden crucifix reappeared on the wall of the village school. Such things were a danger. In order to keep control, it was decreed that all priests must swear a new oath of submission to the laws of the Republic.[15]

Ever since the events of Thermidor 1794, when the tide turned against the more radically egalitarian faction, there had been no restoring of the old certainties. Things had gone too far. The names of things kept being changed, by decree, from Paris. Everyday conversation required a careful pervasive duplicity, according to the convictions and the influence of whoever might be listening. It was all very unsettling. The old and the new names for the days of the week jostled together in the mind. At last, in April 1795, in a pragmatic recognition of the force of popular indifference, the recently decreed obligation to use the Republican decimal calendar for the hours of the day and the days of the week was 'indefinitely suspended'. The rational ten-day week had never been popular.

A vivid local example of this duplicity can be found in the pages of a series of annual almanacs for the Commune of Sens. In the almanac for

Year IV (1795–6), the title page gives only the new Republican calendar and it foregrounds the patriotic phrase 'the Republic one and indivisible'. The next year's almanac, for Year V (1796–7), gives the old-style date in an afterthought. It drops the gesture to the 'one and indivisible', retains the graphic emblem of the sun and reverts to the former street name when identifying the printing house. The street that had been designated rue de la Convention went back to being Grande rue. Likewise, the ebb and flow of collective public emotion was disconcertingly unpredictable. On 28 Germinal Year III/16 April 1795, a local Jacobin, Henri-Marc Desmaisons, was arrested in Sens. Responsible for recent executions, Desmaisons was paraded through the streets to great rejoicing at the humiliation of the *buveur de sang*.[16]

IN THIS CITY, day by day, from the age of eleven until the age of eighteen, in the intervals of reading Voltaire and Buffon and browsing the pages of the *Encyclopédie*, Achille-Cléophas Flaubert witnessed in familiar, local detail a world-historical drama that it would be impossible for him to influence, to understand or to forget. It was an uncomfortable experience, especially for a boy with memories of the judicial persecution suffered so recently by his father. The public events of those years, viewed from the window of a school classroom, offered much to ponder, even for a boy not given to sustained introspection. If Achille-Cléophas had kept any private written record of these early days, he would probably have laid his journal out according to the old pre-revolutionary calendar.

And yet he was quick in other ways to acquire the official language of the hour. It speaks for Achille-Cléophas's precocious resilience that at the beginning of his second school year he was awarded a prize for *morale et bonne conduite*. He was already the ideal student, hard working and gratifyingly receptive. 'His eager nature drove him to seize upon all the treasures of knowledge; he gave himself to the task in hand with all his usual persistence he already gave signs of what he would one day become.'[17]

Promisingly, the youthful Achille-Cléophas did not confine himself, like some dull cartoon bourgeois, to pursuits that were simply useful; there was time and energy for the elegantly superfluous; he was acquiring literary tastes that would endure, surviving even the later pressures of his professional life. His obituary celebrated the fact that 'Monsieur Flaubert was a man of culture; his memories of the classics remained with him down the years and he often added to the charm of our conversation with apt quotations drawn from the authors he had loved in his younger days.'[18]

There is ample confirmation of this eclectic acquisitive habit of mind in the post-mortem inventory of Achille-Cléophas's library. In the year 1846, when an inventory was compiled, his library included works by six major classical authors, all in translation. In terms of quantity, Plutarch in twenty-five volumes and Cicero in thirty-one volumes predominated. The poets Tibullus, Ovid, Seneca and Virgil were there too, but outnumbered. Achille-Cléophas was evidently drawn to Plutarch and Cicero, the exemplary chroniclers and analysts of public life.

When the boy received his first school prize, on 22 September 1796, the college prize ceremony coincided with the celebration of Republic Day. According to local testimony, the staff and the students of the college took part in an early morning procession, from the town hall to the Place de l'Esplanade, where an altar to the fatherland had been set up.[19] Observing all such public events, acutely conscious of the dangers that lay in wait for the impulsive, Achille-Cléophas may have decided that it was wise, in a phrase dear to Stendhal, to hide your life. Best not to have any conspicuous political opinions. Be careful what you say, and don't write down anything that might one day be used against you. The more rigidly righteous of the Monarchists already had a derisive name for all such opportunist survivors. They were ridiculed as weathercocks, *girouettes*, turning with every change in the wind.

Local events pressed heavily upon Achille-Cléophas's first four years at the college. In these years after Thermidor, in this provincial town, there was certainly no sober mood of reconciliation. There was intense, intermittent conflict, simultaneously political, religious and cultural, on the streets, in the churches and in the schools. These were bitter years of recrimination and revenge. There was so much unfinished business, so much damage that had not yet been made good. Someone in every family had a story to tell. In the words of the historian Susan Desan, there was 'an overwhelming political and psychological need to pour out the tragedies of the Terror, to recount personal sufferings and deceptions […] at this moment when the wreckage of human intimacy gripped the social and political imagination.'[20] Achille-Cléophas, precociously attuned to the possibility of sudden misfortune, listens carefully to the stories being told by those around him.

WE MAY PEER INTO THE ENCLOSED WORLD of the college through the window of the prospectus that was published in the local almanac in October 1796. The tone of that document is carefully reassuring. 'Revived' in the autumn of 1795, the college now offers instruction in mathematics, experimental physics, natural history, *belles lettres*, ancient languages, grammar and drawing.

> Citizen Salgues, formerly professeur d'Eloquence, is in charge of the house. Students in his care have available to them individual tutors for Music, Fencing, Dance and Writing. All matters relating to cleanliness, decency and morality are the object of the most careful attention from their tutors. The house allotted to the college is spacious, clean and commodious. Each student occupies a separate room, without however being hidden from the observation of his masters. The food is copious and wholesome. The annual tuition fee is 340 livres, in cash or in kind. Individual tuition in Music, Fencing etc. is paid for separately. Students' laundry and mending is at their own expense. They are expected to provide: a bed, two pairs of sheets, six towels, a plate, a drinking cup, and small items of furniture for their individual rooms. They pay six livres a year to the porter. The Director can nevertheless cover these expenses on payment of a supplement of 25 livres for the bedding, 55 for the laundry and the mending, 120 for individual tuition, or 200 livres for the full complement. The school year begins on 15 brumaire [5 November]; though pupils may be received at any time, and they can be supervised and taught during the vacations if parents so desire.[21]

This syllabus is nicely poised between the old and the new. Frivolous social accomplishments, such as music and fencing, dancing and handwriting, are taught, for a little extra, alongside the sober, bourgeois pursuit of the real, as represented by maths and physics. Achille-Cleophas, true to his origins, would be good at maths and drawing, disciplines of logical sequence, precise measurement and close observation. Fencing and dancing were unlikely to figure among his accomplishments.

The man named as the current director of the college, Citizen Salgues, tutor in experimental physics and natural history, enters our story at this point. Salgues is going to be important. Far from home, transplanted from town to city, Achille-Cléophas was aware that he needed a patron to guide him through this new world. In that recent business with his father, the power of patronage had been decisive. Achille-Cléophas, aiming high, went to the man at the top, the current head of the college. He became a loyal disciple of Citizen Salgues. He kept in contact with Salgues, well beyond his schooldays, frequenting his Paris salon as student and then, in later life, preserving a soothingly idealised and strongly affirmative memory of his old teacher. Salgues was the only thing about the 1790s that Achille-Cléophas cared to remember.

However negative posterity's judgement upon the man and upon the incurably mediocre abundance of his writings, Salgues was a formidably powerful figure in the tense miniature world of the college. Achille-Cléophas took Salgues seriously and thus we need to know who he was, what he did and what notions he might have imparted to this gratifyingly diligent and receptive new boy, the son of that vet from Nogent. Happily, Salgues has left a detailed account of himself.

Writing in the late 1820s, defending himself against the vituperation of his Parisian rivals, Salgues composed a carefully self-justifying political memoir describing his public career during the 1790s. He was now in his seventies, a survivor of the Revolution and still, in his own mind at least, a public figure of some note. Everyone had heard of Salgues. He was the author of a fiercely partisan nine-volume royalist narrative of the events of the Napoleonic era.

The details of Salgues's personal history were soon familiar to his admiring young disciple. Salgues was forty years old when they first met, as master and student, in 1795. For the next ten years, Salgues would be a second father, as well as a source of books and ideas and contacts. He was also, perhaps, a model of how to survive. We shall follow Salgues's history, down through the chaotically eventful years immediately before and after his acquaintance with Achille-Cléophas. As one might expect, it is a tale of heroic moderation sustained all through a decade of blood-stained enthusiasms. For that was how the man saw his own life.

Salgues was born in Sens in 1755, where his father worked as a surgeon, 'exercising the honourable profession of medicine and enjoying a certain public esteem'. Salgues senior was a freemason, one of the founders of a local lodge, Saint-Jean-de-la-Concorde. The family was modestly prosperous:

> And though my father was not rich he sent me to Paris to continue my studies. I prospered there. With a taste for letters and for a peaceful life I entered a career in the church. At twenty-three I was called back to Sens [...] to occupy the chair in eloquence. There I was in contact with the most

distinguished persons of the town. Two princes of the church honoured me with their friendship.[22]

When the Estates General was summoned in 1789, Salgues collaborated on the drafting of the local *cahier de doléances*, the written schedule of grievances being drawn up in every parish. A competent administrator, astute in his cultivation of the friendship of those a little more powerful than himself, Salgues was launched on a brief and stormy career in local politics. In 1790 he was chosen to make the opening speech at the primary electoral meeting. Then he was voted onto the electoral assembly for the department, where he talked down a motion to exclude the clergy and the nobility. Appointed deputy procurator in the new local administration, his first act as a magistrate was an indictment of the fiendish populist Jean-Paul Marat. By the end of that same year he was elected chief procurator in a unanimous vote.

Salgues had already reached the upper limit of his power. 'I endeavoured', he wrote, 'to establish peace and justice within the walls of my native town. Nobody was persecuted for his opinions; the price of bread was easily controlled; and the only oath that ecclesiastics were required to take was the civic oath.' Once again Salgues was nominated elector:

> Had I been ambitious I could easily have been elected to the Legislative Assembly. However I already foresaw the troubles that were threatening us. In 1792, after the unhappy events of 20 June, I went with a deputation from the town of Sens to meet the King and to declare our devotion to his person. That day the men with pikes were in control, and it was easy to foresee what would happen.[23]

In 1792, at some danger to himself, he opposed the decree abolishing the monarchy. In 1793 the local club proposed an address to the Convention, supporting the judgement against the king. Salgues spoke out against it. In August of that same year he refused to implement a decree ordering the imprisonment and deportation of all non-juring priests. He organised a meeting with the authorities to plead their cause as being 'not only the most peaceful but also the most benevolent men'. He was dismissed for his pains, but re-elected within a few days.

His real troubles began in September 1793 when visiting commissioners denounced him to the local revolutionary committee. Three days later, at one in the morning, a group from the committee 'accompanied by armed men' entered his house in order to arrest him. He escaped and went into hiding, 'far from the town'.

The name of Salgues was now added to the list of émigrés. He was effectively an outlaw. For the next five months, all through the autumn and winter of the Terror, he wandered from one hiding place to the next. In April 1794 he came back to Sens, to retrieve his papers. Arrested and imprisoned, he was required to prove, within fifteen days, the fact of his residence in France, on pain of death.

Loyal friends petitioned the Convention on his behalf, and his sentence was repealed. He remained in prison until November 1794. His name was removed from the list of émigrés in the following month. He could soon return to public life. In 1795 he set about rebuilding the local education system, now in ruins, since all the property belonging to the college had been sold off. Salgues began by educating the local children for free, in the very house where he had been imprisoned.

In recognition of this virtuous initiative, he was commissioned to draw up a plan for the colleges in the region. Soon thereafter he was elected head of the restored Collège de Sens, 'on terms most honourable'. He now shunned national politics to concentrate on running the college. The churches in the town had opened for Catholic worship once again, and Salgues was pleased to restore to the cathedral the rich church ornaments that he and the cardinal's librarian had managed to conceal from 'the fanaticism and the rapacity of the revolutionary committees'. After the Vendémiaire rising in October 1795, local Jacobins denounced Salgues for his alleged links with royalist conspirators. Their attack came to nothing. Salgues was safe for the moment.[24]

In 1796, along with two other local notables, he began publishing a newspaper intended to counter the influence of the local Jacobins. In July 1797, emboldened by a royalist election victory, Salgues made the mistake of publishing an invitation to a memorial service in the cathedral 'for the repose of the persons of this town who died during the Terror, victims of tyranny'.[25] A provocative gesture, it must have played a large part in what was about to happen to him. In the wake of the leftist coup of 18 Fructidor Year V/4 September 1797, Salgues was held responsible for a newspaper editorial that was strongly critical of the Directory. The criminal court at Auxerre sentenced him *in absentia* to deportation. Salgues went into hiding for the next eighteen months. Once again, he found that he was listed as an émigré. The college, meanwhile, was handed over to Benoist-Lamothe, an enthusiastic promoter of the novel cult of theophilanthropy.

Exhausted by the miserable life of the fugitive, Salgues eventually gave himself up and was imprisoned. There followed a sequence of successful judicial appeals that were repeatedly blocked by the local commissioner. He finally secured a personal interview with Fouché, the chief of police in Paris. According to Salgues, Fouché recognised the justice of his cause and ensured that all charges against him were dropped. Knowing Salgues's survivalist talent for ingratiating himself, one suspects that this was scarcely the whole story. Did Salgues perhaps purchase his freedom by offering to put his pen at the service of the new regime?

According to his memoir, the year 1800 found Salgues destitute in Paris. He had lost his library, his properties in Sens and his college. In collaboration with two friends from Sens, also refugee moderates, he effected a second reincarnation, this time as an enterprising metropolitan journalist and author of tediously prosaic books of popular philosophy. By the year 1805 Salgues had a salon. Here one might listen in to the fashionable poet in conversation with the fashionable scientist. By 1815 Salgues had earned a prominent entry in Alexis Eymery's *Dictionnaire des girouettes*. Published shortly after the Battle of Waterloo, this was a royalist's satirical revenge on all the opportunists, the survival artists and the 'weathercocks', those men who had turned with every shift in the wind since 1790, refashioning their allegiances whenever necessary. Talleyrand won first prize, awarded twelve weathercocks. Salgues was somewhere in the middle of the list. He had four weathercocks to his name.

4

Reading Voltaire

AFTER THUS FOLLOWING SALGUES FORWARDS IN TIME, we return back to the school year that began in 1797. Achille-Cléophas entered his third year in the autumn. His first two years had been a success. He had found a patron and won a prize. But now, in a dismal repetition of recent events at home, his current patron disappeared. When Salgues was ousted from the college in September 1797, he was soon replaced, at the behest of the administration, by Benoist-Lamothe. Salgues had to go because, unfortunately, in the words of his replacement, 'his principles were not at all in harmony with those of the government, and the municipal administration of this Commune, mindful of the dangers of his influence on the minds of the young, were compelled to remove him from his position as head of the school'.[1]

A man of the same generation as Salgues, Benoist-Lamothe was different from his predecessor in almost every respect. Whereas Salgues, coming from modest artisan origins, had risen in the world by virtue of a scrupulously orthodox intellectual diligence, Benoist-Lamothe was a romantic aristocrat who espoused the cause of the people. If Salgues was the traditional career-creature of the church, Benoist-Lamothe was the new man, a prodigy of virtuous patriotic energy. He came from a noble family; one or two of his close relatives were émigré royalists; he was the exception, the one who had succumbed that mood of generous imaginative exaltation which led to the renunciation of feudal privileges on the night of 4 August 1789.[2] A gentle, congenial and endearingly quixotic character, Benoist-Lamothe was also a fluent maker of verses. Before the Revolution, he had been a provincial celebrity on account of his literary talent; now he was a deist, a disciple of Rousseau and Voltaire, an ardent democrat and possibly a freemason. The patriot–poet, the man with an ode for every occasion, Benoist-Lamothe could turn his hand to anything: speeches, pamphlets, hymns, prayers, dedications and invocations to this or that ideal being.

The political and religious uncertainties of the years 1795–1800 furnished Benoist-Lamothe with a glorious opportunity. The directory was increasingly sympathetic to efforts to harness the formidable power of the religious imagination to the service of the Republic. By the early months of 1797, the new cult of theophilanthropy had emerged as the most successful of the various efforts to cleanse Christianity of its fanaticism. Based on a synthesis of Masonic and Catholic ritual, theophilanthropy was humanitarian and familial, a natural religion that banned all theological discussion and affirmed only two principles: the existence of God and the immortality of the soul. This new cult was suddenly in high favour. With the support of the authorities, theophilanthropists shared the use of church buildings and enjoyed the endorsement of several of the famous names of the day, such as Tom Paine, Bernardin de St Pierre and the painter Jacques-Louis David.

Benoist-Lamothe, soaked in the poetry of the more radical exponents of deism, was the very man for such an adventure of the spirit. Indeed he had already engaged closely with these contentious questions. In the early months of 1796, he published a pamphlet in praise of the Republican festivals, the *fêtes décadaires* instituted by Robespierre. These festivals were still being observed in Sens, though they had largely fallen out of favour elsewhere. They celebrated paternal love, maternal tenderness, filial piety, manhood itself; Benoist-Lamothe was the very man to bring these secular virtues to life. A new religion must fill the cultural space left empty by the elimination of the old. It must: 'Raise altar against altar, reason against superstition, and gradually establish, by mean means of instruction and persuasion, the cult of *la patrie* in place of the vain cult of images, the pure and simple religion of nature in place of the absurd religion of the priests.'[3]

Accordingly, in April 1796, Benoist-Lamothe published in his newspaper an outline account of a patriotic and deist cult, 'Les rites et cérémonies du culte sociale'. Robes and altars, hymns and prayers, bread and candles, all the old symbols could be turned to new purposes. Benoist-Lamothe spoke the language of the hour with an intimidating fluency. Here is an extract from his publication of 1796:

We honour Brutus as the enemy of crowned tyranny, Socrates as the martyr to the truth, Jesus of Nazareth as the first apostle of equality, the honourable victim of Judaic aristocracy and the fanaticism of the Pharisees. […] finally we address our homage, but not our prayers or our wishes, to those glorious martyrs of liberty who have cemented with their blood the foundations of our Republic and have adorned it with their talents and their virtues.[4]

Benoist-Lamothe's *culte sociale* offended the more philosophical patriots as being too flamboyant. After conferring with his fellow theophilanthropists in Paris he agreed to tone it down.

In January 1797, in response to the temporary revival of the 'the absurd religion of the priests', Benoist-Lamothe began publication of a local newspaper, *L'Observateur de l'Yonne*. It ran for several years, promoting the newly minted religion. In September 1797, prompted by the coup of 18 Fructidor, Benoist-Lamothe stepped forward as the local voice of theophilanthropy. His moment had arrived. For the next three years, until Napoleon decreed the suppression of theophilanthropy, the civic culture of the town of Sens was dominated by the new cult.

The town council were sympathetic to theophilanthropy. They gave Benoist-Lamothe the use of the main chapel in the old seminary. The first service in the new temple took place on 21 September 1797. There was a tricolour banner suspended from the ceiling. *Adore God and Love your Neighbour* was inscribed on the wall. The plain altar was decorated with flowers. Accompanied by a group of children, Benoist-Lamothe presided, dressed in white with a purple sash. His initiative was soon rewarded; a second service, a few days later, was well attended by both men and women.

Criticised by local Republicans for retaining too much of Catholic ritual forms, Benoist-Lamothe published a revised edition of his recent anthology of canticles, hymns and odes, cleverly setting the new words to familiar tunes, in order to encourage full participation. The new wine of theophilanthropy tasted better in the good old bottles. Women crowded into the new temple, wearing their cherished religious trinkets. By the end of December, such was the success of the new cult that they moved the services into the local Cathedral of St Stephen. Both the town council and the commissioner attended the inaugural service there, acclaiming it as a great victory over the local Catholic faction, with whom they shared the use of the building. The Catholics, for their part, deplored their rivals' use of the choir. It was pollution. They insisted on reconsecrating the cathedral each time they came to use it. But the theophilanthropists were in the ascendant. Locally, they outnumbered Catholics.[5]

In addition to his leadership of the civic cult, Benoist-Lamothe was newly installed as the head of the college. In October 1797 he published a rousing educational manifesto in the pages of the local almanac. A triumphant appeal to the citizens of Sens, it is of great interest for what it tells us of the new dispensation under which Achille-Cléophas was to spend the later years of his time at school in Sens. Here Benoist-Lamothe dispatches Salgues, his predecessor, with a powerfully vague narrative of recent events.

> Public education, which had been neglected for some years in the Commune of Sens, had come back to life. Friends of Literature all applauded the energy and the ability of the man [Salgues] who happily presided over this restoration of public education. But unfortunately since his principles were not at all in harmony with those of the government, the municipal administration of this Commune, mindful of the dangers of his influence on the minds of the young, were compelled to remove him from his position as head of the school. With him there fell that valuable institution which was beginning to flourish under his leadership. But thanks to the zeal of the municipal administration, thanks to the good will and the public spirit of certain men of letters who are keen to work alongside us, the moment has come to rebuild the temple of the arts in this Commune.

He follows this with clever play on the theme of individual ambition:

> Citizens, the arena of Letters will be open once again on 1 Brumaire this year. Would you be so heedless as to fail to enrol your children? Because there are no ecclesiastical sinecures for them, do you think that there is no point in making educated men of them? A deplorable error which, if it is not promptly vanquished, may cause incalculable harm both to the Republic and to yourselves! Consider! Are your children not destined impartially to become the administrators, the magistrates, the legislators, perhaps even the governors of the future? And do you think that an ignorant man could proficiently occupy any position of such importance? Even electors and local officials require a certain education and knowledge. A day will come, have no doubt, when public office will only be open to those who can give

proof of having followed a course of study in one of the central schools, or at least a secondary school. May this our wish be heard and understood and embodied in law by the representatives of the Nation![6]

WE DO NOT KNOW what Achille-Cléophas made of the sustained local enthusiasm for theophilanthropy during these proverbially receptive years of his early youth. Watched over as they were for positive signs of patriotic emotion, it was probably unwise for any aspiring boy of fifteen or sixteen to appear openly indifferent. In later life Achille-Cléophas appears cautiously neutral towards the church. He did not publically criticise religious belief; on the wards of the Hôtel-Dieu he worked alongside nuns who provided most of the nursing care; in his personal library there were no religious texts of any kind.

If Benoist-Lamothe and theophilanthropy left no permanent traces in Achille-Cléophas's imagination, this may be thanks to Voltaire. At some point, before he left Sens for Paris, while he still had time for extra-curricular reading, Achille-Cléophas began reading Voltaire. There is a good chance that he began with a little portable volume of thirty sous, the pocket-sized 1769 edition of Voltaire's *Philosophical Dictionary*.

The preface of that work offered an irresistibly amusing invitation to join an elite of urbane and enlightened persons.

> The book does not demand a continuous reading; but at whatever place you open it, you will find something to think about. Those books are most useful in which the readers do half the work themselves; they develop the thought whose germ has been presented to them; they correct what seems defective, and with their own reflections strengthen what appears weak. This book will be read by enlightened persons alone; the common herd are not made for such knowledge; philosophy will never be their portion. […] the common people do not read; they work six days a week and go to the tavern on the seventh.[7]

To read Voltaire, at a tenderly receptive age, was to imagine for oneself, however belatedly, however youthfully and provincially, the intellectual liberty of the Enlightenment, that liberty which Kant defines as 'emergence from our self-imposed immaturity'. Voltaire was amusing, playful and sardonic, and yet that fierce comic spirit was gainfully employed in coaxing one to attend to the more demanding ideas that figured on the curriculum of modernity. In the words of Peter Gay, Voltaire

> pointed to Locke, champion of philosophical modesty, empirical inquiry, and associationist psychology; to Newton, enemy of vain hypotheses and creator of the true system of nature; to Hume, philosophical unmasker of miracles, penetrating psychologist, and natural historian of religion. […] If we do not, and cannot, know the essence of things […] we will not persecute others, who are as ignorant as we are. Thus scientific method and religious toleration, Newtonian physics and the attack on fanaticism, are aspects of a single enterprise.[8]

In the words of Achille-Cléophas's first biographer, 'he shaped his youthful mind by reading the mocking philosopher'.[9] From this simple statement, there arises a nicely elusive question. What did it mean, for Achille-Cléophas, to *read* Voltaire? More precisely, to read him at the age of sixteen, in the year 1800, in the town of Sens?

It's worth noting that Voltaire is the only serious author named in Achille-Cléophas's obituary. Buffon is not mentioned. Neither is Rousseau. (Had he been reading *La Nouvelle Héloise*, rather than *Candide*, he might have emerged a different man.) Observe that he didn't just 'read' Voltaire, he 'shaped his youthful mind' by reading him. The French idiom is distinctive: *élever sa jeunesse*. The verb means to raise, in the sense of to form, educate, shape, train. Among all the other books he remembered, Voltaire was the most important.

At around the age of sixteen, then, we may say that Achille-Cléophas was uniquely receptive to the lesson of Voltaire. He used those texts and he made them his own. He was possessed. Imaginatively, he became Voltaire; he became like the man whom he imagined as the source of the texts that he was reading. Reading Voltaire was irrevocable, an initiation, something never to be repeated with any other author.

The boy read his Voltaire, and the man thereafter cultivated a Voltairean persona. Voltaire was immediately useful: it was a name, a style of thinking, a habit of mind that consecrated the boy's dawning sense of his intellectual superiority. The message from Voltaire was thrillingly sombre. It said: stop wandering in a dream. Observe the world that awaits you. You must see things, as they are, if you hope to make your way in such a world. Otherwise you will drift along, powerless and bewildered.

In a world still so slow and heavy, so stubbornly, so lamentably ignorant, let your thoughts run swift and light.

How did this happen? Who put him onto Voltaire? It was unlikely to have been Salgues. For all that his father was a freemason, Salgues was vigorously pro-clerical in his political sympathies. In the good old days, before the Revolution, Salgues had been the dependable houseguest of the local bishop. In these hard times, Salgues was the loyal defender of the church. He surely had no time for the man who jokingly styled himself Beelzebub's theologian. Benoist-Lamothe, Salgues's successor as head of the college from the autumn of 1797, is the most likely source of Achille-Cléophas's abiding attachment to Voltaire. Theophilanthropists greatly admired the mocking philosopher for his assault on superstition.

But which Voltaire did they admire? The *Collected Works*, published in the late 1790s, ran to seventy volumes. Surely, this was an embarrassment of riches. Such abundance was overwhelming. It needed sifting and sorting, if it was to be of any use. For the educated citizen-patriot of 1790, the question was what should we do with our hero Voltaire to show our gratitude?

By the summer of 1791, an answer had been found. For the second anniversary of the fall of the Bastille, Voltaire's remains were disinterred from the graveyard of the abbey of Scellières, where they had reposed for the thirteen years since his death. They transported the remains, with full ceremony, from the site of the Bastille, through the streets of Paris, to the Pantheon. On the platform bearing the coffin, there were three inscriptions. They describe in brief how Voltaire was imagined in the years after his death. The first inscription said: 'He avenged Calas, La Barre, Sirven and Monbailli.' The second inscription said: 'Poet, philosopher, historian, he gave a great impetus to the human spirit and prepared us to be free.' The third inscription said: 'He combated atheists and fanatics. He inspired tolerance. He reclaimed the rights of man against serfdom and feudalism.'

Those inscriptions testify, forcefully and confidently, to the liberating powers of the written word in the hands of the heroic ethical subject. Much had happened since 1791 to tarnish one's optimism. Several heroic ethical subjects had been led to the guillotine. Be that as it may, nine years later, in 1800, at the age of sixteen, in a town still dominated by theophilanthropists, to encounter Voltaire was to participate in an exhilarating rite of intellectual emancipation.

Voltaire made very good sense, in the light of all that Achille-Cléophas had already experienced in recent years. He taught a lesson of comic resilience. He fortified the mind against the harsh and puzzling features of the adult public world: the adversity, the injustice, the fanaticism, the oppression, the violence, the sudden loss of the things one loves, the gleeful malice of the powerful. He also taught a lesson of resistance. He inspired faith in the adversarial powers of reason, a bold integrity in the face of oppression and injustice, an integrity that found expression in mordant satire. If you survived the 1790s, Voltaire was your ideal mentor.

Achille-Cléophas perfected a combative Voltairean tone. The imitation was so successful that a certain imperious irony became the native habit of his mind. The effect on those around him, both family and colleagues, was formidable and disconcerting. According to Védie, colleague and biographer, Achille-Cléophas preserved a certain heroic singularity:

> His indifference to what are called honours led him to criticise those of his colleagues who only believe in their own talents when they can enhance the sound of their names with some impressive-sounding qualification, and he used to denounce, with an enthusiasm that was both charming and acerbic those who spent their days not in deserving their honours but in scheming for them.
>
> In this regard he had a certain affinity with Voltaire. In fact he had indeed educated his youthful mind by sustained reading of the mocking philosopher. […] And one came across that keen and penetrating gaze, as well as that mocking smile, so nimble and so searching, which is the hallmark of a mind given to satire.[10]

That 'keen and penetrating gaze' was a memorable feature. Achille-Cléophas had a look that Gustave Flaubert would later compare to the action of a scalpel. To be looked at, by father, in one of his darker moods, was to undergo a form of moral vivisection.

FOR SUCH A BOY, in such a time and place, Voltaire was a useful intellectual hero, and Achille-Cléophas was not alone in his choice. For the liberal elite of this generation, Voltaireanism was a powerfully congenial structure of feeling. The theoretical nuance deserves some emphasis. To quote Raymond Williams's definition, the concept of a structure of feeling is chosen 'to emphasize a distinction from more formal concepts of "world-view" or "ideology". [...] We are talking about characteristic elements of impulse, restraint and tone; specifically affective elements of consciousness and relationships: not feeling against thought, but thought as felt and feeling as thought.'[11]

For Achille-Cléophas, Voltaireanism was no mere youthful affectation. It became the habit of a lifetime. The 1846 post-mortem inventory of his library mentions an edition of Voltaire in seventy-two volumes.[12] Though we do not know the year in which Achille-Cléophas acquired his Voltaire, the fact of its presence in his library confirms both the consistency and the intensity of his attachment.

To own a complete Voltaire, especially in the years before 1830, was to make a muted political gesture of dissent. During the reign of Louis XVIII (1814–24) Voltaire's complete works, published in lavish 75–100 volume sets, became bestsellers. Anxious to register their dissatisfaction with the new regime's proximity to the church, wealthy anti-clericals subscribed in great numbers. Between 1817 and 1830, much to the dismay of the church hierarchy, no fewer than twenty-one separate editions of the complete works were undertaken. One and a half million volumes of Voltaire were printed.[13] One's edition of Voltaire was intended, in equal measure, for social display, for bemused contemplation and for reading.

That Voltairean pose of sardonic amusement was an agreeably versatile mode of feeling. It could always be happily married to an essential benevolence. In the 1790s, it could fortify the mind of an ambitious boy who found himself cast adrift, like a later version of Candide, in a world governed by capricious acts of violence. In the years after the Restoration, when the public sphere was being purged of atheists and radicals, the Voltairean attitude allowed a man of humane liberal sympathies to indulge among trusted friends in superior and consoling forms of philosophical laughter.

Ever alert to the insufficiencies of those around him, Achille-Cléophas Flaubert remained, resolutely but prudently, the child of an earlier, more enlightened, more sceptical age. After 1815 he would encounter professionally a new generation of compliant Catholic monarchist colleagues, privileged mediocrities with friends in high places, men such as his detested junior colleague Dr Hellis. In such situations, Voltaireanism was a great comfort. It allowed one to castigate all things sentimental, romantic and religiose. It affirmed a heroic lucidity, untainted by the new fashion for the adoration of things ecclesiastical and monarchical.

This version of the Voltairean emerged, I suggest, only in the 1790s. It fitted the everyday experiences of the literate, modernising, scientific elite who were hoping to do well out of the new order of things. It equipped them, affectively and rhetorically, for the tedious conflict with the unenlightened, a term that encompassed devout, ignorant peasants who believed in magic, as well as stubborn Catholic royalists who believed that one day everything would be restored to them. Elite Voltaireanism evolved as part of the complex political culture of the day. After 1815 it probably served to protect and preserve some remnant of the heroic optimism of the immediately preceding generation, that mood of militant futurity represented so powerfully in Condorcet's text of 1795, *Esquisse d'un tableau historique des progrès de l'esprit humain.*

VOLTAIRE COULD BE OPENLY AFFIRMED. Other loyalties may have been more problematic. There is a possibility that either Salgues or Benoist-Lamothe may have initiated Achille-Cléophas, informally, into the ideas and the ideals of freemasonry. Benoist-Lamothe is the more obvious candidate, though Salgues turns out to be the more likely. As already mentioned, it is evident from the local archives that Salgues father, a surgeon practising in Sens in the 1790s, was a freemason. Salgues senior is named as one of the founders of a local lodge, Saint-Jean-de-la-Concorde, in a document from 1777. The fact that Salgues senior was a surgeon may also be significant. He may have suggested to Achille-Cléophas the possibility of his studying surgery; although that idea may have come simultaneously from Achille-Cléophas's maternal grandfather who was also a surgeon.

On the other hand, if Achille-Cléophas Flaubert had remained a freemason, this would have been evident from the 1825 police report compiled to investigate his political opinions and activities. Perhaps Achille-Cléophas was a freemason at some point during the First Empire, either in Paris or in Rouen. It is worth mentioning that as a student in Paris, he was in contact with several of the eminent scientists of the day, men such as the geographer Alexander von Humboldt, to whom he gave anatomy lessons, and the chemist Louis Jacques Thénard, in whose laboratory he worked as an assistant.[14] These men were likely to have been freemasons, though it must be observed that Achille-Cléophas's contact with them was not sustained beyond his Paris student days.

Highly influential among urban professional elites, freemasonry was the object of hostile official scrutiny in the years after the fall of Napoleon. According to the modern historian Sudhir Hazareesingh, 'In 1825 the prefect of police, in a detailed report on conspiratorial activity among French Freemasons, even asserted that masonic endeavour was "republican in nature" […] Lodges were places where men could discuss ideas of freedom, independence, constitutionalism, and above all irreligion.'[15] If Achille-Cléophas had ever been drawn towards masonic circles, he later covered his tracks with some skill. A youthful enthusiasm, a mildly embarrassing memory; masonry would clearly be too contentious a thing for a man in his position.

5

Parisians

Paris is the centre of the science of medicine and the chosen land of those dedicated to its pursuit. It became his home, as soon as he realised what facilities for study it offers; the emulation it inspires; the encouragement it provides.

— XAVIER BICHAT, *Essai sur Desault* (1798)

ACCORDING TO THE REVOLUTIONARY CALENDAR, an awkward contraption that one used to advertise one's enduring loyalty to the slightly tarnished idea of the Republic, 1800 was Year VIII of Liberty. On 12 Messidor, Year VIII, Nicolas Flaubert wrote to the citizen sub-prefect of the Department of the Aube, petitioning the administration for funds to support the further education of his talented son, Achille-Cléophas. That document is worth quoting in full. It's a decorous specimen of patriotic republican discourse, and it gives details of the recent family history of the petitioner.

Liberty Equality
To the Citizen Sub-prefect of the Commune of Nogent-sur-Seine
Nicolas Flaubert, veterinary artist, of Nogent-sur-Seine. *Declares* that, for the last four years, he has exhausted all his resources in order to fund the education of his son, now aged fifteen and half, and to make him a useful member of society; that this son is already well versed in the complexities of mathematics and of drawing; as well as in the other primary sciences which are the basis of solid understanding; that it would be miserable for him to see wasted all the money which he has struggled to find, right down to the

present day, a thing which will come about, by reason of the losses which he has sustained from his modest fortune, over several years; if the government does not come to his assistance by granting his son free admission either to the Veterinary School at Alfort or to the École polytechnique. He therefore begs you, Citizen Sub-prefect, on the strength of the information to which you have access, and on the basis of this statement, to support his request and to urge it on the government. To do so would be an act of justice, and would be to render a great service to a father who always does his utmost to be of service to his fellow citizens by his art.[1]

In particular, what are we to make of that muted complaint at recent difficulties: 'the losses which he has sustained from his modest fortune, over several years'. Behind that wary reticence, there is the fact of Nicolas Flaubert's recent prison sentence. Perhaps, since his release, there had been no more lucrative government contracts. Even so, parental ambition on behalf of the son had not been relinquished; the money needed to keep Achille-Cléophas at the Collège de Sens had somehow been scraped together; the money to send him on to the next stage, to Paris, would likewise be found.

The petition must have been successful, even though Achille-Cléophas did not pursue either of the two possibilities, Alfort or the École polytechnique, that his father had envisaged for him. What happened next is best told in the words of Caroline Commainville, writing a family history at a distance of some seventy years: 'The situation of the family was very modest; nevertheless, with great effort, they sent him to Paris, to study medicine.'[2]

Achille-Cléophas arrives in Paris early in November 1802, Brumaire Year IX, new style. In the national mind, if only in the well-fed, propertied and enfranchised portion of that mind, the Revolution is finally and blessedly over. The man of the hour, First Consul Bonaparte, has said as much. The evidence is everywhere. The churches have been unlocked. The priests are returning. The old Gregorian calendar, once reviled as a monument of servitude and ignorance, has now been restored to respectability. Elegant decimal watches, their dials inscribed with rational tens and hundreds, were once the conspicuous emblems of the affluent patriot. They are no longer the fashion. If you still possess one, these days, you will probably leave it at home. Bonaparte has decreed that the ten-day Republican week, the *décade*, is henceforth suspended for government employees. Sundays can once again be taken as a day of rest. The old names for the days of the week can once again be spoken aloud, without fear of criticism from some zealous, snooping neighbour. They say that the Revolution is over, but who knows what comes next?

ACHILLE-CLÉOPHAS WAS ABOUT TO BE EIGHTEEN when he arrived in Paris to begin his new life as a medical student. This was a moment to remember. In later years he would describe this chapter of his life, more than once, with discreet satisfaction, to deferential junior colleagues. He was young, he was ambitious, he was bright and he was in Paris. 'My only patrimony', he would say, looking back, 'was my intelligence.' An aspiring student from a modestly successful provincial family, he was, like many others, travelling light. Though we may confidently surmise that he carried with him the Paris address of his old mentor, Citizen Jacques Barthelmy Salgues. The chameleon priest had evolved once more. Now he took the stage as the metropolitan jack-of-all-trades author and salon host. For a young man on the make, Salgues would be a useful contact. Even in a strenuous Republic of Virtue, for such it still claimed to be, mentors were to be cherished.

Apart from such schoolboy attachments, Achille-Cléophas also carried one large though invisible burden: the expectations of his modest, self-sacrificing, loyal, provincial family. He would long remember that they had saved for years to send him to Paris. He was there in the name of the family. He must make the most of their gift. Work hard. Never falter. Never deviate. Such thoughts, imperiously repeated to oneself, beget a habit of single-minded persistence. Friends will call this quality of his character by various names: tenacity, fortitude and resilience. Rivals may call it something less admiring. The latter, obliged to tolerate his brisk, cheerful, habitual superiority, may ask each other if the man liked to exaggerate the modesty of his family of origin. It made his success seem all the more miraculous. Be that as it may, all such mellow pleasures in the story of his early years were still far away in the future. The young student had arrived in the great city and must now make his way in the world.

THE WAR WAS OVER and November 1802 was a most auspicious moment for any youth to enter the turbulent flow of the national life. In March of that year, the Treaty of Amiens had at last ended the war between France and Britain. That war had dragged on for ten years; it had impoverished both nations; it had imposed on both French citizens and British subjects a deviously authoritarian political culture. The war was over, for the moment at least, and the general mood of the hour, as expressed on the streets and in the drinking-shops of Paris, was triumphantly festive.

Certain proscribed persons, such as priests and aristocrats, could now be cautiously welcomed back into the body politic. Priests had indeed reappeared miraculously from the shadows, reinstated in return for an oath of allegiance. Easter Sunday 1802 saw the first official Easter celebration for ten years; Bonaparte used this occasion to announce an amnesty for the majority of those émigré aristocrats who were still loitering in exile beyond the frontiers of the Republic. Sceptical spirits were already wondering apprehensively where might be the limits to the powers of young General Bonaparte. Would he be content to remain First Consul? Did he have further ambitions? Perhaps it was already too late to ask those questions. In July of that year, in high places, there was loose talk of the restoration of Empire. 'Bonaparte,' they said in London, 'is supposed to have taken Charlemagne for his model [...] a plan that is calculated to dazzle the people of France, and to flatter their vanity.'[3]

In the mind of the newly arrived Achille-Cléophas, there were no such dissenting thoughts. How could a young man not be dazzled? Bonaparte, at this moment, was the supremely good thing. There is evidence for Achille-Cléophas's enduring admiration for Napoleon. It is teasingly fragmentary but convincingly miscellaneous. There are three suggestive items. The first was displayed in the main dining room of the house at Croisset in 1846, a portrait engraving of Napoleon, 'in a gold frame, value fifteen francs'.[4] The second such item was to be found among the books in Achille-Cléophas's study in 1846. The postmortem inventory lists *Mémoires de Napoléon* in eight volumes, meaning the series of texts published in years just after Napoleon's death in 1821 by two of his companions in exile, Gorgaud and Montholon. Their full generic title was *Mémoires pour servir à l'histoire de France, sous le règne de Napoléon, écrits à Sainte-Hélène, sous sa dictée, par les généraux qui ont partagé sa captivité.* That running title was abbreviated in the page headers to *Mémoires de Napoléon.* In the study at Croisset these eight volumes of memoirs were shelved, strangely, in among books otherwise exclusively on physics, chemistry and medicine.

What do we make of this anomaly? Judging from the sequence of titles in the inventory, the shelving of all the books was carefully thematic. The memory of Napoleon is nesting in among the emblems of Achille-Cléophas's highest professional ambitions. This fits with the third item of evidence. In the obituary pamphlet of 1847, Bonaparte is described as 'the consular genius who [...] wished to inflame every heart with a fiery spirit of emulation'.[5] This is the exalted idiom of Republican virtue, marvellously insulated, after so many years, from any ironic reappraisal. It captures the youthful mood of 1802, as well as the mature but still untarnished memory of the fifty-odd months of the Consular period (December 1799 to May 1804) that saw Napoleon's rise to power. *Fiery spirit of emulation*: what better way to dignify the memory of one's youthful ambitions? Every emergent bourgeois meritocracy will thus drape itself in some happily resonant phrase copied from the warrior epics encountered in the schoolroom.

Meanwhile, all through the summer and the autumn of 1802, crowds of English visitors made their way to Napoleon's Paris. Safe passage to France had been impossible, ever since 1793. Ten years of aggressively patriotic anti-French satire had done their best to protect the loyal British intelligence from the seductions of republicanism. That danger was over. Now that the road to the continent was open once again, people of fashion, as well as people of ideas, were eager to see for themselves what had become of the beloved national enemy. In Paris, there would be something for every taste:

> Politicians were anxious to study the new government and its head. Soldiers were curious to see Bonaparte and his victorious legions. Artists embraced the opportunity, by so short a journey, of inspecting the spoils of Italy collected at the Louvre. Men of letters and science were desirous of consulting documents or of forming or renewing acquaintance with French celebrities. Clergymen went to see whether Catholicism had really recovered its sway after the eclipse of the Terror. Bankers and merchants were eager to recover confiscated property and old debts, or to revive business relations.[6]

In that summer of 1802, the thirty-two-year-old First Consul, General Bonaparte, could still plausibly be regarded as the friend of liberty. The younger sort were mostly still natural Bonapartists. William Hazlitt, currently in the city with a commission to copy the Italian paintings in the Louvre, was a great admirer and would remain so, perhaps beyond the limits of any rational attachment. The awkward imperial meta-morphosis was politically imminent, in the name of continuity and stability. Friends of liberty might not approve, but one day very soon, Bonaparte would be emperor. Emboldened by the August plebiscite that confirmed him as First Consul, he amended the constitution and became absolute monarch in all but name. He was henceforth to be known as Napoleon, rather than Bonaparte.

THE LINEAMENTS OF that Napoleonic world-transforming energy – yet to be labelled as bourgeois individualism – may already be faintly visible upon the still-boyish face of Achille-Cléophas as he looks out, at last, on the city that is now to be the first great theatre of his ambitions. The social world of the Republic of 1802 was no longer dominated by hereditary privilege. The reformed medical profession offered the perfect opportu-nity for advancement. A qualified physician could usually avoid military service; now that many of the old elite had disappeared from the scene, a young man might rise quickly to a position of profit and power. Ever since the coup d'état three years previously, First Consul Bonaparte had promoted his new men. The beneficiaries quoted that clever phrase of his: 'la carrière ouverte aux talents'. A powerful slogan, it spoke to persons of intelligence and energy. Loosely translated, it meant 'I can go as far as my talents will take me'. In 1802 it also implied something else: no need to worry, these days, about that cumbersome Jacobin doctrine of equality.

Achille-Cléophas spent the next four years of his life, the supremely receptive years, in Napoleon's Paris. He was lucky to be there, at the heart of the action, during the good years, the years before the high cost of being seduced by Napoleon became evident from the casualty lists.

The immediate signs of the times were generally propitious. With the coming of peace, the streets of the capital were now crowded with masons and carpenters. After ten years of wartime neglect, public build-ings were being repaired and beautified. Three new bridges were being built over the Seine. Whole streets were being pulled down for rebuilding. The marks of devastation were being removed from the churches, those that had not been converted to shops and warehouses.

The 'English Visitor' of the London *Morning Chronicle*, ever critical of all things French, observed all this worthy endeavour with a nicely measured disdain. 'It is easy to conceive', he wrote, 'that Bonaparte should wish to do all this from the well known magnificence of his views; but how he is able to supply the expense appears altogether unaccountable.'[7]

The great city itself was an education in the imminent pleasures of modernity. Places of public amusement were constantly crowded. The English Visitor further observed that 'all ranks seem to have a sort of horror of being at home'. This is oddly to their credit, for 'It is not the custom, as in England, to sit four or five hours after dinner, drinking to intoxication, and rendering themselves incapable of any rational enjoyment.'[8]

Along with his fellow citizens, Achille-Cléophas could witness the rational marvel of the *thermolampe*, the first gaslight in the world. This recent invention drew great crowds to the rue Saint Dominique, where the inventor charged three francs for admission to a memorable display. The Visitor reported diligently that

> Citizen Lebon, an engineer, is able, for twenty-four hours, to spread, throughout seven large apartments, the mildest heat and the most vivid light, and, at the same time, to enlighten a large garden in such a manner as to make it appear like noon-day. The flame can be shown detached from all support, and can be modelled to any shape. When enclosed in a crystal globe, the flame by no means soils it.[9]

The harsh brilliance of the gas-powered *thermolampe* dazzled eyes that had previously only ever beheld candlelight, firelight and the glow of the oil-lamp. The *thermolampe* was the new Enlightenment, the practical triumph of vision, reason and science. Consciousness itself was about to be configured to a new rhythm. Gaslight was liberation from the ancient tyranny of the dark, but it was also a disenchantment of the night, obliterating the stars. Gaslight would make possible urban 'nightlife', citizens strolling in safety along well-lit streets; it would also intensify the exploitation of labour, allowing expensive factory machinery to work around the clock, no longer confined to the hours of daylight.

Every young man from the provinces, however tightly purposeful, pauses to admire the shopping arcades, 'a recent invention of industrial luxury [...] glass-roofed, marble-panelled corridors extending through whole blocks of buildings [...]. Lining both sides of these corridors, which get their light from above, are the most elegant shops [...].'[10] By 1802, in the city of Paris, there was already a choice of arcades. The Passage de Caire, the very first arcade, had been built in 1799 on the site of the garden of a former convent. Amusingly, the arcade was paved with recycled grave-stones, their inscriptions still intact. The sphinx-like stone heads over the street entrance to the Passage de Caire were a nice touch. Commercially astute and irreproachably patriotic, they celebrated Bonaparte's recent triumphant return from Egypt.[11] The rival Passage des Panoramas enticed the stroller with two rotundas where panoramic views representing the landscapes of large cities were projected.

As well as the gas-lamps, the arcades and the panoramas, Paris offered rational enjoyments of a more elevated kind. On the south bank of the Seine, by the Pont d'Austerlitz, there stood the great botanical garden, the Jardin des Plantes, formerly known as the Jardin du Roi. Recently renamed and augmented with a menagerie, it now housed a great collection of sci-entific books harvested from the libraries of émigré royalists. Originally a garden full of medicinal plants, open to the public since 1640, the Jardin des Plantes was a spacious urban park, laid out with rectilinear severity. Full of trees and flowers and paths for strolling, the garden also offered the citizen the pleasures of a labyrinth and a maze as well as the menagerie.

Unlike many of the principal cultural assets of the Ancien Régime, the garden had survived the Revolution. Indeed it was cherished as an object of national utility. It was a virtuous enterprise that would, in the resonant words of the politician-scientist Antoine-François Fourcroy, 'seek to bring together all the knowledge and all the objects of service to the progress of the natural sciences, and consequently to the progress of agriculture and medicine, commerce and the arts.'[12] In addition to its boundless intellectual utility, the garden would also be a moral inspira-tion, an embodiment of those Enlightenment ideals propagated by the heroic polymath-curator of the previous generation: Buffon.

Georges Louis Leclerc, comte de Buffon (1707–1788), mathematician, cosmologist and naturalist, was the author of a literary enterprise that paralleled the *Encyclopédie* of Diderot. He was the author of the thirty-six-volume *Histoire naturelle, générale et particulière* and also curator of the Jardin du Roi for nearly fifty years, from 1739 until his death in 1788. In that capacity, he transformed the place from an apothecary's garden into one of the centres of European science; he recruited many of the best minds of the rising generation; he doubled the area of the garden to nearly eighty acres, by acquiring various adjacent parcels of land. In the mind of its new management, Buffon's garden figured as a living symbol of the highest ambition of the Revolution: to regenerate the nation.

Achille-Cléophas, recalling the elaborate botanical flora once compiled by his father, understood this garden and the powerful ideas of perfectibility that it embodied. To have read the *Histoire naturelle* was to have the mind prepared for those great themes of liberty and regeneration by Buffon's distinctive lyrical mix of philosophical argument and sublime images.[13] Reading Buffon was a potently sensuous apprenticeship to the principal ideas of the Enlightenment. As one appreciative contemporary reader expressed it:

> [...] his reasonings and inferences are not only bold and ingenious, but adorned with all the beauties of expression and all the charms of novelty. They everywhere lead to reflections which are momentous and interesting. They expand the mind and banish prejudices. They create an elevation of thought and cherish an ardour of inquiry. They open many great and delightful prospects of the economy of Nature [...].[14]

Achille-Cléophas's personal library would one day include an edition of Buffon in 127 volumes, alongside his editions of Voltaire, Rousseau and Condillac. That edition of Buffon was complemented by the presence of the works of Erasmus Darwin and of Lamarck. As his early biographer put it, Achille-Cléophas 'combined the study of medicine with the study of the other sciences'.[15] Judging from the later contents of his library, Achille-Cléophas was a man who preserved a sober intellectual passion for the great scientific ideas of his youth. We may picture him, then, the solitary delighted nineteen-year-old student strolling the alleyways of the Jardin des Plantes on a winter morning early in the year 1803. In a singular piece of indulgence, he has just purchased – and he will soon be reading – a recently published book by the garden's professor of zoology, Jean-Baptiste Lamarck. There he will encounter a most interesting new word: *biology*.

ON THE STREETS OF PARIS, just outside the utopian garden, the national imagination is beset by anxiety. Conspiracy, surveillance, espionage and assassination: these are the sombre themes of well-informed conversation. The English Visitor observes that

[...] alarmed for the safety of the new political fabric which they have, with so much curious labour, and with such high promises, reared. [...] the public mind is [...] not at all in a state auspicious to the duration of the present government; and [...] the people think much more of the burdens of taxation [...] than of the splendid schemes which the First Consul is so zealous to advance.[16]

In the radical coffee houses, it is said, in a cautious undertone, among those who make it their business to know about such things, that there will soon be a scheme to deport 'all who are obnoxious to Bonaparte, to wander among the wilds of Louisiana, or to perish under the torrid heats of Cayenne'.[17]

Walking the streets, or parading the public gardens, the Visitor duly observes 'the perpetual recurrence of the military uniform, and the [...] disgusting surveillance of the bayonet'. 'Every coffee house, every restaurateur, every place of general resort [...] contains spies of the police. [...] When you begin to speak freely of politics in a public room [...] a Frenchman draws himself up with a sort of anxiety and fearfulness almost comic.' 'It is treating Frenchmen like lunatics, who even in their lucid intervals must not be allowed to go abroad without their keeper and the instruments of coercion.'[18]

The official language of the hour strains credulity in its heroic efforts to drown out all such unspoken thoughts of danger. The Visitor relays the following ripe specimen of Napoleonica to his London audience: Proclamation from the Prefect of the Lower Seine, to the Citizens of Rouen, announcing the imminent arrival of the First Consul.

It is to him you are indebted for victory, for peace, for the return of morality, order and law; it is he [...] who devotes every moment of his life to your prosperity. The name of the hero fills the world. Foreigners hasten to contemplate him from the ends of the Earth. Everywhere, within, without, his words have been received as the oracles of wisdom; he is become the common arbiter of people and kings.[19]

The truth of all this was not yet apparent to the general population, exhausted by the war and now briefly bedazzled by the promises of peace. The First Consul was energetically refashioning the Republic to suit his darker political purposes. In the words of Chaptal, the newly appointed

Minister of the Interior, this was the moment to 'recreate the unity of the French […] and reinforce the authority of the Republic'.

The symbolic powers of the Catholic religion were especially useful in soothing from the collective imagination all those persistent and troubling memories of violence. Ambitious young men discover that it is prudent to be seen attending Mass. You keep quiet about your atheism, if you want to get on in the world. Chateaubriand's *Génie du christianisme* (1802), an exalted celebration of the poetry of Christianity, perfectly caught that mood of general yearning for the restoration of all the good old things that the nation had supposedly lost since 1789.

6

The New Science of Man

The present epoch is one of those great periods of history towards which posterity will often turn its gaze, and posterity will hold to account all those of us who could have hastened and assisted the progress of the human race along the road of improvement.

— XAVIER BICHAT, *Essai sur Desault* (1798)

CHATEAUBRIAND WAS INTENT on discrediting the ideologues. That new word, *idéologues*, concealed an old heresy. Chateaubriand deplored their godless conception of man as a material organism in which the physical and the moral faculties are inextricably confused. Such profane, materialist speculations were mischievously destroying the foundations of religious faith by denying the ancient promise of the immortality of the soul. It disheartened submissive paupers who trusted in the afterlife, as well as soldiers required to die for their country. In the de-Christianising 1790s, Enlightenment materialists, positioned near the centres of state power, had enjoyed a brief ascendancy. Now, in 1802, as the priests returned and the churches were restored, these same materialists were in retreat. This was not a good moment for conspicuous intellectual audacity.

What was a young medical student to do? The old quarrel between science and religion would not be resolved within Achille-Cléophas's lifetime. Reading Voltaire had cleared the ground. But what was to be cultivated there now, upon that invitingly empty cultural terrain, in place of superstition, in place of crimes committed in the name of reason and virtue? What did one read next, after reading Voltaire?

Two names came most readily to the fore. The aspiring youth must read Cabanis and Bichat. Although they were already of the older generation, their books were recently published and their ideas remained appealingly but discreetly contentious. Collectively, their writings defined the possibility of a modern medical science grounded in the new conception of how the body and the mind, how the physical and the moral might be reconciled. Cabanis, and Bichat, taken together, offered something irresistible: theory and practice harmonised, human happiness augmented. At the very least, human misery reduced.

AMONG HISTORIANS, it is generally agreed that the foundations of modern clinical medicine were laid here in Paris around the year 1800. Though the details remain a matter of debate, it is further agreed that clinical medicine in its modern form grew out of the late Enlightenment vision of a new science of man. That new science, it was hoped, would fulfil the ancient Delphic injunction, *know thyself*. Man, regarded as an object of science, would be restored to his place, in nature; human reason could then be liberated from the ancient tyranny of the supernatural. In the light of the new science, the physical and the mental, so long split apart by superstition, would now disclose their true unity, 'confounded at their source', according to Cabanis's memorable phrase.

There might be no limit to human power. Would *that* be entirely a good thing? Such gloomy questions would have to wait. Regardless of whether we now regard the science of man as covertly authoritarian or as unambiguously benevolent, the original promise, however tentative the fulfilment may have been, spoke persuasively to the young medical student who had arrived, so recently and so eagerly, at the centre of things.

We know what Achille-Cléophas brought with him, intellectually, to his medical training. We know what he read at school, and we have some idea what he made of it. Voltaire and Buffon, both recently deceased, offered an admirable apprenticeship. The former exemplified the power of individual reason; the latter celebrated the minute observation of the real. After clearing away the superstitious rubbish of the ages, where did Enlightenment lead? And, more to the point, how long would it take a young man to get there? By a nice coincidence, in 1784, the very year that Achille-Cléophas was born, Kant had defined Enlightenment as 'man's emergence from his self-imposed immaturity'.

Having made it to Paris, increasingly aware of his superior powers, enthralled by the imperatives of metropolitan intellectual emulation, Achille-Cléophas was ready for that next step. He was, of course, lucidly and unswervingly ambitious. That quality was woven into him, by paternal example; and by the political culture of the hour. He would become an inclusive man of science, as well as merely a physician. 'Just as he had won first prize in all subjects at College, so he combined the study of medicine with that of the accessory sciences.'[1]

The most influential living representative of the new science was Georges Cabanis (1757–1808). Cabanis was a trained physician, a man of refined philosophical and literary interests; he was also a versatile political survival-artist and a formidably proficient intellectual entrepreneur, endowed with practical energy and supported by powerful allies. From the early years he had been a judiciously moderate Republican and a friend of the Revolution. A man of many parts, he had been successively physician to Mirabeau, a hospital reformer, the editor of Condorcet's papers, author of many official papers and reports, a member of the Council of 500, and latterly a co-conspirator in Bonaparte's coup of 1799. In his idle moments, Cabanis worked on the great project of his youth, a verse translation of *The Iliad*. By 1801, critical of Bonaparte's authoritarian policies, and enfeebled by his own declining health, he had resolved to absent himself from public life. He would now concentrate on publishing his scientific writings.

It was most instructive, for any youthful admirer, to contemplate the early career of Citizen Cabanis. This was evidently how it used to be done, before the Revolution. Impeccably well connected, Cabanis *came up* rapidly, as a very young man, through the usual metropolitan networks of patronage. In his early twenties he frequented the great salon of Madame Helvétius. Installed as her youthful favourite, he lived as a perpetual house-guest, at her villa, out in the suburb of Auteuil. There he encountered many of the best minds of the late Enlightenment: D'Alembert, Condorcet, Chamfort, Volney, Marmontel and Diderot. The talk in that illustrious circle was memorably anti-clerical, reformist and favourable to the American Revolution.

Like so many of his kind, Cabanis was also a freemason. From his early twenties he was a member of the Loge des neuf sœurs, where he met many of his future ideologue associates. A cautious, freethinking, liberal elite, the lodge brothers neglected masonic ritual in favour of cultural and scientific discussion; they admitted women to meetings; they supported humanitarian ideals, including benevolence to the poor and universal brotherhood. Playing safe, they refrained from speaking against religion, morality or the state.[2] It was not yet time for radical talk to venture out beyond the confines of the salon and into places where it might make mischief.

When the salon talk of the 1780s became the public policy of the 1790s, George Cabanis, now in his mid-thirties, was well placed to contribute to that exhilarating national political conversation. Married to Condorcet's widow, Cabanis was administrator of hospitals, professor of hygiene and then professor of legal medicine. In 1802, with all this behind him, Cabanis published his major work, a review of the natural sciences, entitled *Rapports du physique et du moral de l'homme*. A substantial compilation in two volumes, the book brought together the series of twelve lectures that Cabanis had once delivered, in rather different times, from the centre of the official culture of the Republic, from the platform of the Class of Moral and Political Sciences at the National Institute in 1796–7.

By the year 1802, that sustaining institutional context, along with the attendant Directoire mood of optimism, was already a thing of the past. Bonaparte was about to clip the wings of the surviving *philosophes*, gathered so conveniently in their Parisian enclave, the Class of Moral and Political Sciences. He did not approve of the ideologues, those idea-mongers, with their belief in observation and experiment and the powers of reason.[3] Their contentious, critical blend of empiricist epistemology, monist metaphysics and liberal politics was too much for a First Consul keen to restore general social harmony. One knew exactly what that sort of thing could lead to. Their platform could not be demolished, but it could, let us say, be lowered.[4]

As a veteran of many committees, Cabanis had a clear sense of what the age demanded. Prudently, he removed traces of the original Republican rhetoric of 1796 from the book that he published in 1802. Comparing a series of quotations from Cabanis praising the medical vocation, we can appreciate the skill with which he covered his tracks. Writing in 1795, with an official commission to sketch out a plan for the reform of medical education, Cabanis ended his four-hundred-page survey of the field with a peroration in the high Republican style of the hour:

And we, dedicated to the relief of human suffering, so often holding in our hands those interests that are most dear to the heart of man; we whom the importance of those interests obliges to seek enlightenment in all quarters, we whose studies embrace nearly the whole range of knowledge both physical and moral: shall we alone be exempt from the right to serve the whole human race, by our efforts, and to contribute to its progress? No, certainly not. Let us be united in our efforts: let us bring to the study and the practice of our art, that philosophy and that superior reason without which, far from providing useful help, our art often turns into a public menace. Let us dare to forge new links between medicine and the other parts of human knowledge. Let knowledge benefit anew from the connection. And at this time when the French nation is consolidating its Republican existence, let medicine, thus coming of age, enter into a new era of its own, rich both in individual glory and in the general welfare.[5]

The spirit of heroic futurity, so compellingly embodied in Condorcet, speaks out once again through Cabanis. Three years later, writing in 1798, reporting to the Commission for Public Instruction, Cabanis strikes a note equally positive, though rhetorically more sober:

> Linked at innumerable points to most of the other sciences, medicine has strongly reflected this movement of regeneration. Already its teaching and its clinical methods have assumed a new character. The philosophical spirit of the century begins to give it both greater ambition and greater precision.[6]

By 1802, four years later, the pursuit of health and happiness, notions decorously vague, has replaced the more fiery Republican language of regeneration and glory.

> The study of the physical man is of equal interest to the physician and to the moralist; it is almost equally necessary to both. Uncovering the secrets of the organism, observing the phenomena of life, the physician endeavours to ascertain what makes for a state of perfect health; what factors may disturb that balance, by what means it can be preserved or restored. The moralist strives to grasp the more obscure operations that constitute the functions of the intelligence and the actions of the will. He is seeking the rules that should govern life and the roads that lead to happiness.[7]

Much of the original intellectual audacity had survived by going underground, buried deep within the text, rather than being paraded, vulnerably conspicuous, near the beginning or the end. Cabanis's insistence on the unity of the physical and the mental was certainly an affront to any orthodox Catholic of 1802. In this newly conceived material world, all is matter and motion. There are no capricious spirits to confuse, and to enchant. If there is no soul then there is no immortality and no afterlife; thus, if one is consistent, there is no good reason to revere the supposedly sacred person of the king. Cabanis concedes that these are 'issues that have never been debated with impunity'. Reader, be warned. 'You will not find here any of what has long been called *metaphysics*: these are merely physiological inquiries'.[8]

In keeping with his new tactics of obliquity, Cabanis waits several hundred pages before he springs the following nicely ingenious surprise on his readers. The brain, he argues quite innocently, is an organ that produces thought. Then the provocation comes, in the choice of analogy. It is obvious, he says, that just as the stomach and the intestines digest food, so the brain 'digests' impressions and then 'secretes' thought.[9] It was the mischievous choice of 'secretes' that gave Cabanis's analogy its mildly scandalous currency later in the coming century. A generation later, in his polemic against all the bad new things, *Signs of the Times* (1830), Thomas Carlyle decried Cabanis's description of the brain. It was, argued Carlyle, a symptom of the creeping power of mechanistic thinking. It was perhaps sobering to consider, in 1830, how the great secular vision of human regeneration had faded, to reveal only the harsh reality of the factory system and its noxious effects on public health.

None of that historic bathos was evident to the young man who opened the pages of the newly published volumes of Cabanis in 1802. We may say with some confidence that Achille-Cléophas read Cabanis, and that he was influenced by what he read. His personal library eventually included a two-volume edition of Cabanis's *Rapports du physique et du moral de l'homme*. The presence of that book testifies to the energy, the breadth and the duration of Achille-Cléophas's intellectual interests, beyond the immediate requirements of his clinical work.

But a more elusive question remains. Which portions of Cabanis did Achille-Cléophas make his own? Which of those ideas did he find congenial, and what did he do with them? I have noticed one idea in particular. It appears in Cabanis and then eventually, smoothed and sanctified by repetition, it becomes a Flaubert family proverb. Colloquially, it says that habit dulls both pleasure and pain. We may call it Cabanis's Law, the law of diminishing sorrow.

It was of course a widely accepted physiological principle that sensations, both painful and pleasurable, fade with the passage of time. Achille-Cléophas refers to this in his 1808 lectures on physiology: 'The senses, sight, hearing, the vocal and the locomotive organs, the intellectual faculties, none of these can be continuously in action. Habitual sensation blunts feeling. Reflection, imagination cannot be always in motion.'[10] This idea had an illustrious pedigree. Bichat picked up the idea from Cabanis, he in turn attributed it to Condillac, and he traced it back to Locke. Cabanis expresses it thus: 'It is an invariable law of animate nature [...] impressions that are too intense, too often repeated, or too numerous, become weaker [...] the faculty of feeling has limits that cannot be violated.'[11]

This was a useful idea for a surgeon, and for the family of a surgeon, obliged to eat and sleep and dream in uncomfortable proximity to all the clamorous fear and pain that was unfolding adjacent to the very room where they took their meals. Reassuringly, Cabanis's Law made some sense of the chaotic intensity of the emotions one was witnessing, every day, in a hospital where surgical operations were conducted without anaesthetic. It offered a medical perspective, cool but not heartless, on those emotions. One knew that their very intensity guaranteed their transience. There are no eternal sorrows and that is a physiological fact. Cabanis has said so.

This is a recurrent theme in Gustave Flaubert's letters. Here it is, for instance, in a letter to Louise Colet, dated 2 September 1846: 'Even the tightest knots come undone on their own, because the rope wears out. Everything goes. Everything passes away, water flows – and the heart forgets.'[12] A received idea; Gustave received it, at an early age, from his father. It promises that emotion, however imperious, is fugitive. This 'physiological fact' legitimates a tough-minded, manly detachment from all that suffering. It allows you to observe, to describe and to understand. Thus fortified, the surgeon can operate. Thus reassured, the novelist can narrate and his endings will deny the violence of the tragic by dwelling instead upon the mild, insidious erosion of desire and identity that the years will always bring. The endings of both *Madame Bovary* and *Sentimental Education* both obey this law of diminishing sorrow. Flaubert's refusal to contrive a consolingly conventional happy ending provoked his contemporary critics beyond measure. Such heartless lucidity, decried as realism, provoked a scandal.

ALONGSIDE CABANIS, in the autumn of 1802, the more enterprising medical students were reading Bichat. The late departed, the much lamented Xavier Bichat was one of the most talented and eloquent medical scientists of the day. Like Mozart, he had done great work at a prodigiously early age. Still in his twenties, Bichat had rewritten the basic principles of physiology. On 22 July 1802, Bichat died of meningitis, worn out by sleepless nights, intellectual work and long hours in the amphitheatre. He was only thirty.

On the day of Bichat's death, one of his prize students dissected the master's body; such was the dispassionate custom of the profession. He noted 'an occipital skull fracture', probably a consequence of the meningitis that had been the cause of death. Secretly, or perhaps with the collusion of one or two fellow-students, the young disciple then severed the head from the body, took it away, boiled it up, stripped it down, and hid it away for the next forty years. Only in 1845, at an official ceremony to move Bichat's remains to the cemetery of Père Lachaise, was the skull reunited with the body from which it had been surreptitiously detached.[13]

Contemplating this choice medical anecdote, we are struck by the theme of affiliation. In the mind of the disciple, Bichat's head is the repository of a secret power that can be conserved and hoarded away. Medical knowledge, according to this belief, is not acquired purely by rational, intellectual effort. Because medical knowledge involves repeated transgressions, it partakes of the magical; it is inherited, as well as acquired. Knowledge and authority are imparted, with a high charge of affect, from master to pupil, as if from father to son. This made for relations of patronage, discipleship, and fraternal rivalry that were often problematic.

The events of the Revolution complicated this peculiar problem of affiliation and patronage. In Paris in the year 1802, the scientific community was struggling to consolidate itself, after ten years of disruption and uncertainty. The old Academy of Sciences had been abolished in 1793 and its members had soon been dispersed by the Terror. The fortunate ones either fled the country or went into hiding. The unfortunate were imprisoned or executed. By 1795, the worst being over, patrons and protégés could once again seek each other out. For the survivors, though, the game had changed. The older generation was often divided by recriminations and rumours on the dangerous question of who had done exactly what during the Terror. Depleted in numbers, in energy and in morale, the older generation was now unusually dependent upon the young who had, in many instances, rescued them from persecution and imprisonment.[14]

Bichat *came up* at just this moment. His whole career was, of course, the subject of ceaseless professional gossip, envious and admiring in equal measure. For many of those who came up soon after, the life of Bichat exemplified the pattern of contemporary scientific ambition. In this diffuse and impersonal sense, Bichat was Achille-Cléophas's elective precursor. When Achille-Cléophas read Bichat, along with the text he assimilated the legend that already surrounded the illustrious name. In the fanciful heroic idiom of official memory, Bichat's genius was like a meteor crossing the sky or a torch that burnt out all too soon.[15] The mix of science and magic was irresistible. In a decisive imaginary act of affiliation, Achille-Cléophas elected to be one of the children of Bichat.

This confident hypothesis rests upon two pieces of evidence. The first is the simple textual fact of Achille-Cléophas's quoting from Bichat in the lectures on physiology that he gave during his early years in Rouen. The second is a more complex literary fact. Gustave Flaubert, when imagining medical greatness, for the closing pages of *Madame Bovary*, conjures up the compound figure of one Dr Larivière. This imaginary doctor is closely based on a real doctor, Gustave's father. According to *Madame Bovary*, Dr Larivière/Achille-Cléophas 'belonged to the great school of surgery that sprang from under the apron of Bichat, to that generation, now extinct, of enlightened physicians who, cherishing their art with fanatical passion, exercised it with exaltation and sagacity.'

There is a significant textual detail in this passage that is often lost in translation: *la grande école chirurgicale sortie du tablier de Bichat*. They sprang from *under Bichat's apron*. The apron is of course the protective leather garment worn in the dissecting rooms of the early nineteenth century. The notion that Bichat's followers sprang out from under his apron is a nice, mock-epic, mythological touch. It also suggests that one's relationship to Bichat might have a richly affective, symbolic dimension to it, an unwieldy psychological fact best acknowledged in the form of a joke. The enlightened physician, both passionate and sagacious, is a most attractive ideal. In the fictional world of *Madame Bovary*, uniformly blighted by intellectual mediocrity, Larivière is the only character endowed with any real creativity. The aggressive side of his genius finds expression in an urbane ability to play on words, undetected by all those around him, the creatures of a lesser world.

The posthumous image of Bichat, youthful genius struck down at the height of his powers, added a compelling magical supplement to the emergent science of physiology. To that image, potent in its simplicity, we must now add a brief account of the real Bichat, if we are to take the measure of the man and to establish what he meant to the generation who came immediately after him. The very disjunction between the life and the legend will have much to tell us about the vocation of medicine in the early years of the new century. It will be argued that Bichat's superbly eloquent account of the medical vocation was his way of confronting a recent political history that remained unspeakable. Out of that confrontation, from under Bichat's apron, as it were, a new structure of feeling emerged.

Born in 1771, Bichat was going to be, for better or for worse, a child of the Revolution. And yet, the events of that Revolution appear to have left no trace in his writings. His recent biographer Elizabeth Haigh found 'no reference to political events in any extant work or letter composed by Bichat.'[16] She suggests that he did this in order to spare his family any anxiety concerning his safety. The truth of Bichat's reticence was probably rather more complex. Though there are only fleeting references to political events, the exalted style of the Republican vanguard permeates Bichat's writings. His writing is implicitly and insistently politicised at the rhetorical level. More elusively, it is also politicised at the figurative level. For example, Bichat's eerie physiological definition of life as 'the ensemble of functions that resist death' encapsulates an anxious psychodrama in which the fragile organism endlessly *resists* all the powers of dissolution that lie in wait, everywhere, out there, in that hostile world. French neoclassical painting of this period often celebrates precisely such terminal scenes: great men dying surrounded by their disciples, the human community barely surviving the endless attrition.

The son of a country physician, Bichat displayed a precocious interest in science. The boy set about dissecting cats and dogs at the age of seven, so it was said. If all had gone according to plan, Bichat would have studied at the medical school in Montpellier, like his father, and then taken up medical practice somewhere in the tranquil rural hinterlands of

the Rhone valley. The Revolution thwarted all such expectations. In the
early months of 1791, on a quixotically egalitarian impulse, the National
Assembly voted to abolish formal medical education, along with many
other remnants of corporate privilege. Anyone who paid the licence fee
could now practise medicine. In that year, at the age of twenty, Bichat was
apprenticed to Marc-Antoine Petit, chief surgeon at the Hôtel-Dieu in the
city of Lyon. Remarkably, Petit was only six years older than Bichat. This
was a fact that any aspiring subordinate would find encouraging. Bichat
was soon conscripted, along with other medical personnel, to help deal
with the health crisis caused by the war with Austria and Prussia. The
improvised military medical service was in disarray. 'The roads leading
back into France from Belgium and the Rhineland were littered with dead
horses and broken or mired hospital wagons. Fleeing health officers carried away their bags of equipment or left them behind to be broken open
and scattered by pillagers.'[17]

In this state of emergency, with no formal qualifications, Bichat found
work as a surgeon's assistant in the hospital hurriedly set up in the seminary where, not so long ago, he had been a schoolboy. Here was a world
in which familiar things – such as one's school – kept abruptly changing
into other things. Momentarily, it gave an enlivening sense of possibility, though eventually it led to a certain numbness. One day, there might
be time to explore the psychological effects of all the violence inflicted,
endured or merely witnessed during the Revolution. This was not yet the
moment. Perhaps a young surgeon such as Bichat was better equipped
than most to live with jumbled memories of bodies in pieces.

By the summer of 1793, the nation itself was in pieces. In the cities
of the south and the west, Jacobins were being guillotined, hanged or
drowned by vengeful crowds in revenge for their more recent virtuous
crimes. There was street fighting in Lyon. A local alliance of royalists and
moderates rose up against the municipal authorities and beheaded the
ex-mayor. In May, the city seceded from the Republic. A militia of ten
thousand men, under the command of a royalist officer, took control of
the city and began preparations for the inevitable counter-attack. Xavier
Bichat was there, a pair of hands, helping to build up the city's defences.

In July, the Republican Army of the Alps, ten thousand men under
General Kellerman, arrived at the city walls. They came with heavy artillery and an ultimatum. All persons not citizens of Lyon were to leave
immediately, on pain of being regarded as conspirators and enemies of

the people. Accordingly, on 1 August 1793, Bichat left Lyon and returned home to the village of Poncin.

There was very little respite. In September 1793, Bichat was once again drafted into the military medical service, caring for wounded troops from the siege of Lyon, the siege from which he had escaped. In December, he returned home, to find that his family was in trouble. Local radicals were accusing his father, formerly a deputy of the Third Estate, of *incivisme*, that dangerously vague offence. To clear the family name, Bichat enrolled for service in military ambulances. Once again, he had been deflected by the Revolution. Once again, he was required to improvise.

Battlefield surgery, then as now, was a primitive business. In 1793, the French military surgeon carried a standard-issue black Morocco box divided into compartments. The black box contained bandages, tourniquets, sutures, needles, a probe, tweezers, scissors and forceps, along with a scalpel, the leaf-shaped blade riveted to a bone handle, and a crescent-shaped amputation knife. In his coat pocket, to comfort the wounded, the surgeon also carried a small leather bottle of sweet spirits of wine.[18]

Extricating himself from the vindictive and capricious drama of local politics, Bichat eventually made his way to Paris. Here he might resume his medical education, if he were allowed into the city itself. When he arrives at the Porte d'Orléans, on 30 June 1794, he must show the militiaman his *certificat de civisme*. This is the new internal passport, a precious document issued only to individuals of proven patriotism. The city itself is in a state of high collective anxiety. The Terror is at its height. Danton was guillotined less than three weeks ago and Robespierre now has slightly less than a month before he too will be dispatched to meet the Supreme Being of his imagination. The tavern talk is all of conspiracies, real and imagined. The harvest is still many weeks away and the price of bread is rising.

As well as that *certificat de civisme*, Bichat was also probably carrying a letter of introduction from Marc-Antoine Petit, surgeon of Lyon, to one Antoine Desault, surgeon of Paris, and Petit's former teacher. Despite all the uncertainties of the hour, the informal system of medical patronage was working quietly, linking the generations and ensuring the transmission of cultural authority, even at such a time, when all such transactions were frowned upon in the name of transparency.

Bichat was taking a risk, attaching himself to this new mentor. Illustrious and influential though he was, Desault had a history. He had antagonised the patriots by his intransigent air of superiority. It was rumoured that he was a royalist. True or not, it might be unwise, in these uncertain times, to associate with such a man. In these circumstances, persecuted by an ignorant and ungrateful world, Desault was delighted to find in Bichat a perfectly loyal and supremely talented young disciple.

Within a few months of arriving in Paris, Bichat had so impressed Desault that the older man adopted him, as both his co-worker and as a member of his household. This arrangement, so gratifying to both parties, lasted less than a year. In June 1795, Desault died of a fever. It was said, here and there, that he had been poisoned, in revenge for his recent role as one of the physicians caring for the Dauphin, the child Capet then languishing in prison. Desault, so it was said, had refused to acquiesce in a plot to murder the child.

Bichat was twenty-four years old when his mentor died. He attended the autopsy, and noted its findings in some detail. He then set about the task of editing Desault's unpublished research papers in anatomy. This richly symbolic sequence, this father-and-son drama of succession, was characteristic of the surgical profession. The master leaves his body to be opened up and meticulously dissected by his apprentices. Accordingly, Bichat witnessed the undoing, the surgical dismemberment of the body of the beloved master. He watched the opening of the skull. He examined its contents. He observed the remarkable depth of the convolutions, the dull colour and the extreme softness of the grey matter. After this dissolution, there followed a figurative restoration, editing and publishing Desault's papers, a labour of love that secured the master's intellectual legacy.

Bichat's obituary for Desault is a fine specimen of the formal public eulogy then customary within the profession. But it is also a compelling meditation on the theme of the medical vocation in the years immediately after the Terror. Perfectly fluent in the exalted, imperative Republican idiom of the day, Bichat delineates the emergent ethos of the enlightened physician, *le médecin-philosophe*. Here was something noble that might yet be salvaged from all the violence and the misery. In the few years left to him, Bichat's writings expound their rapturous theme: the growth of the physician's mind as he fulfils the heroic quest for knowledge.

Achille-Cléophas read these texts by Bichat, at some point during his Paris years. Beyond their various rhetorical occasions, they add up to a young man's manifesto for a new medicine. Woven into its rational substance, the new medicine offers an exalted professional ethos, a new structure of feeling perfectly fashioned to the demands of this historical moment.

According to Bichat, the century of wonders has just begun, and the way into the future is wide open. The enlightened physician shall carry forward the promise, the vision and the idealism of the Revolution, purified of the destructive malevolence of politics.

> Passionate about our art, eager to acquire new knowledge, to make new discoveries, we would compel all the human sciences to pay a proper tribute to Medicine. And thus, we love *belles lettres*, because they can deck with flowers a knowledge [*science*] of such sublimity and splendour, knowledge whose eternal charms have all too often been profaned by a crude philosophy. We love moral philosophy, because without it we have only a clumsy, imperfect, material knowledge of man. We love physics, because we are ourselves one element in the great system of the world, and without it we would be condemned to know nothing of what lies all around us, and nothing of ourselves. We love chemistry because it obliges nature to take us into her confidence, to show us her secrets and her deepest mysteries. We love natural history; in a word, we love universal philosophy, because we are convinced that any medical theory will be wise and well-founded insofar as it can identify itself more intimately with the general science of relations, something of which practical medicine is merely the corollary or application.[19]

Achille-Cléophas's inaugural speech to the Rouen Academy in 1815 will affirm Bichat's vision. It will lack something of that youthful audacity, though it will be more richly nuanced.

7

Anatomy Lessons

Great minds live, mostly, in the hope that their names will never die, and nearly all of them die without having lived for another. They covet honour and they spurn pleasure. One might say that as their intelligence grows and spreads, so their souls shrink and turn inwards.

— XAVIER BICHAT, *Essai sur Desault* (1798)

WHEN ACHILLE-CLÉOPHAS ARRIVED in Paris, the senior medical establishment, depleted by the vagaries of political persecution, was especially receptive to incoming new disciples. For these few years, the path to the top would be clear. Even so, the life of a medical student was not easy. The years of newly codified medical training were expensive. In 1800 it could cost about 5,000 francs. Then you might have to find another thousand francs to pay a substitute to do your military service.[1] Every year over a thousand students enrolled to study medicine in Paris and they were all in fierce competition with one another.[2]

In this professional jungle, Achille-Cléophas prevailed, as he was accustomed to do, by the simple force of intelligence and hard work. At the end of his first year he won first prize and had his fees rescinded. For three years in a row he won first prize at the prestigious École Pratique. It was a conspicuous success and it entitled him to have his fees paid by the state.[3] For all that, he had a hard time of it. Achille-Cléophas caught tuberculosis during his first winter in Paris.

Medical students were vulnerable. They lived in great poverty. They wore shabby clothes, they ate a meagre diet and they lived in cold, dismal rooms. Most of them wore cheap wooden clogs rather than shoes.

According to a contemporary prospectus, the medical student could expect to work a fourteen-hour day. From six until half past eight in the morning surgeon and students make the rounds of all hospital patients. From nine until eleven practical surgical lessons are held in the hospital amphitheatre. From eleven until three, there follows an intensive sequence. There are outpatient consultations; presentation of hospital patients; operations to be performed on that day, with discussion and demonstration on a corpse; anatomical examination of deceased patients; reports on patients previously operated on; remarks on the character of illnesses then prevalent in hospital; thorough discussion of one disease selected for attention that day. Participation by students was required at each step. At three o'clock, there is the anatomy lesson. The surgeon questions the students on the previous day's lesson. At four thirty, the students go to the patients' rooms for dressings. At six o'clock, students reassemble in the amphitheatre for further outpatient consultations. At each point, students will engage in practical exercises: making dissections, practising operations on corpses, making up equipment, applying bandages.

> The course is heavily practical in aim and methods. The goal is to produce competent practising surgeons by immersing students in routine clinical observation and treatment, giving them daily exposure to surgical technique and human anatomy. Instruction and examination is oral and practical rather than written and theoretical. The student learns by seeing and doing. For all of this the hospital locale is decisive. Steady turnover of a large number of patients presenting a variety of diseases, opportunity for clinical study and regular autopsy of a relatively large number of cases, amphitheatre doubling as a classroom and as an operating room, separate from the wards, ready availability of rooms for dissection and dissection material, these conditions come together only in the institutional context of the hospital.[4]

Achille-Cléophas now needed to acquire the practical knowledge of anatomy that could only be had, one slice at a time, in the dissection room. In Paris, there was an abundant supply of the essential materials, especially during a freezing winter.[5] Dissection would be one of Achille-Cléophas's favourite pursuits, an intellectual passion he continued to cultivate far beyond the requirements of his profession. Habitually, according to his colleagues, Achille-Cléophas spent 'entire nights spent in the dissection room, his favourite pursuit in a life so severe and so determined'.[6] Such prolonged obsessive labours eventually damaged his health, so they said. In a more positive vein, Gustave Flaubert recalled 'his father at the age of sixty, on a Sunday, a fine summer day, telling his wife he was going for a walk in the country and then slipping out through the back door, running off to the mortuary and dissecting as though he were still a medical student'.[7] Gustave also carried less happy childhood memories of spying upon his father engaged in dissecting a female corpse. On this occasion though, he was trying to impress his new lover, Louise Colet, with the message that he had 'seen everything', long ago.

Little could ever be done to veil the hideously repulsive side of anatomical dissection. In the 1820s, Charles Darwin abandoned his Edinburgh medical studies in disgust at this abhorrent professional necessity.[8] The invention of refrigeration and the publication of *Grey's Anatomy* would greatly alleviate – though it would not eliminate – the bloody practicalities. Meanwhile, in the early years of the nineteenth century, in any city where medicine was taught, there was always a certain dark trade in corpses. Recently departed criminals and paupers, cumbersome, putrefying fragments of mortality, were procured legally or illegally, transported openly or covertly, and then, after dissection, somehow they were disposed of, decorously or not. The whole secret business of the dissection room was inevitably the perennial object of popular horror and official concern. Every citizen was uneasily aware of the source of a certain filthy smell that assailed the senses somewhere on the less affluent streets of their city. According to the contemporary theory of disease, that smell, that *miasma*, was also a fearful source of infection.

Such was the practice, repellent and transgressive. According to the theory, anatomy was noble and virtuous. It was a heroic quest for material truth as well as a revelation of divine order. According to the 1751 edition of the *Encyclopédie*, that compendium of Enlightenment values,

> The human body is a machine subject to the laws of Mechanics, Statics, Hydraulics and Optics. [...] You have to open up a few corpses, peruse the vital organs, delve among the entrails [...] those who have not ventured into the labyrinth of *Anatomy* are not worthy to enter the sanctuary of Medicine.[9]

Lest this jittery ambivalence be too uncomfortable, there was thankfully a way for both deists and atheists to agree on the instructive purpose of the inevitable desecration of the corpse. The *Encyclopédie* argued that

> The human body is one of the most beautiful machines to leave the hands of the Creator. Self-knowledge assumes knowledge of the body, and knowledge of the body assumes knowledge of such a prodigious constellation of causes and effects that it must lead directly to the notion of an intelligence both wise and omnipotent. Such knowledge is, so to speak, the very foundation of natural Theology.[10]

The strangely assorted idiom of this passage suggests a muted cultural anxiety. The register keeps shifting: the prosaic artisan, delving and perusing, becomes the romance hero, conquering the terrors of the labyrinth and winning his way into the sanctuary. The flawlessly Newtonian machine-thing is also a sublime testimony to the intelligence of the Creator.

If the theory was confused, the practice remained loathsome. Medical students were notorious, detested by the common people for their criminality. Their misdeeds were common knowledge. Students would attack the site of an execution to remove the coveted fresh corpse. They would steal corpses from the common graveyards where they lay in ditches, great layers of them, twenty deep. They would bribe the gravediggers, or pay local prostitutes to create a diversion while they lifted the cadavers, conveying them four or five at a time in a *fiacre*. The police mostly turned a blind eye to it all. The students would hide the corpses and dissect them furtively in the attic of some house in the cheapest, poorest part of the city. The sequel was no less reprehensible. In Paris, on the city dump out at Montfaucon, half-dissected human heads and miscellaneous body parts were often found among the sewage. The students disposed of the bits they couldn't incinerate on the spot by dropping them into the nearest sewer pipe.

In late eighteenth-century Paris, on the place Maubert, the medical entrepreneur Desault – a man we have already encountered in relation to his pupil Bichat – had the first amphitheatre for dissection. His initiative yielded a good profit. By 1803, there were fifteen amphitheatres in the city. Prompted by complaints about the smell, and by the knowledge that existing regulations were largely ignored, an Ordinance from the prefect of police set out comprehensive new regulations.

From the details, we can reconstruct the things that were not supposed to be happening. Unlicensed anatomy theatres on inappropriate sites were henceforth forbidden. Premises must be fumigated every day and dissections must only take place in the five colder months, from November to March. There was to be no dissection of corpses with contagious diseases. Cadavers were to be transported decorously in covered wagons. During dissection, canvas screens were to be set up to block the view from neighbouring windows where young women might gather to look on. Debris was to be removed every day, rather then every ten days.

In the last days of Napoleon, a great medical scandal came to light. It confirmed all the most lurid popular suspicions about the anatomists. A circle of dissection room employees had been making big money by secretly selling off vast quantities of human fat to the local enamel workshops. Animal fat, human or equine, produces a high temperature flame with almost no residue. For this reason, animal fat commanded a high price. Two thousand litres of human fat were found, hidden away in the dwelling of an employee of the medical school. For fear of alarming the public and possibly causing a riot, the case was tried in secret. All of the accused were sentenced to six months in prison. At the request of the Faculty of Medicine, delinquent employees were merely cautioned.

There was general surprise that this illicit trade had never been noticed before. Employees had always been perfectly open about it. They collected and melted the substance down on the premises of the Faculty. Selling on the fat was simply one of their cherished perquisites. In 1810, at the time of Napoleon's marriage to Marie Louise of Austria, the fat-traders had done exceptionally good business, selling carnival lanterns that burnt with a suspiciously bright flame.

An official report published a generation later, in 1831, in the newly established journal of public health *Annales d'hygiene publique et de médecine légale*, deplored with much eloquent detail a range of enduring abuses.

> Many amphitheatres had neither courtyards, nor sumps nor drains for the liquids; some were located in houses so dilapidated that the staircases were dangerous. It was a sport and so to speak a point of honour to defy the police, to ignore the regulations and provoke the inspectors. The windows were always open, and the canvas screens placed in front of them were either torn or missing; they unloaded the carts that brought the cadavers in

the street, often in broad daylight, and similarly they took away the putrid remains; ordinarily the cart was left all day in the street at the door of the amphitheatre, announcing by the smell it gave off the uses to which it was put. In several places they threw all manner of debris down into a small yard, from third- or fourth-storey windows, leaving the walls impregnated and impossible to clean.[11]

Anatomists were not indifferent to the emotions that assail the practitioner in search of the truths of the body. It could be argued that for the young anatomist of the year 1802, the emotions prompted by the practice of dissection were more distressing than those typically experienced by the medical student of a generation earlier. With the demise of natural philosophy as the framework for the investigation of life, with the consequent indifference to the question of the soul, with the secularisation of scientific knowledge, the practice of anatomy had very recently lost its old restorative quality of sacred ritual. According to historian Andrew Cunningham, 'Anatomising no longer illustrated the wisdom of the Creator [...] only the complexity of the organisation of the organism.'[12] The modern anatomist may be in perfect control, technically, but he is also silently struggling with compulsive intimations of nothingness.

> The appearance of the lifeless man, the difficulties, the horror and the danger of the dissection, the careful inspection of all body parts, the enveloping silence which seems to disclose to the spirit the nothingness of the matter to which it is attached by an invisible thread, over which it has power, these things repel most of those who have to do with the vast array of human infirmity.

That was written in 1819 by a colleague of Achille-Cléophas. The theme of horror and nothingness, intruding here upon an otherwise conventional eulogy for a colleague recently deceased, is promptly banished by means of an ambiguous gesture that evokes an older, residual, religious context.

> The friend of science, the friend of man, ignores all such impediments. His senses seem impassive in the midst of this lugubrious scene; nothing intimates to him that he himself could be attacked by our common enemy at the very moment when he is about to take hold of his secret and push back the limits of his power. He sees only marvels, he feels only admiration and the hope of being useful, and his mind and his heart are equally satisfied.[13]

Here, within the confines of a single sentence, we can detect something of the unresolved contemporary debate between religion and science. *In extremis*, the man of science standing alone at the dissecting table will feel as if he is under attack from 'our common enemy'. In that anxious moment, he must convinces himself anew that he is doing good. And so he reaches out for the old ethos of natural philosophy, 'he sees only marvels, he feels only admiration'.

AS ALREADY MENTIONED, during his first winter in Paris, Achille-Cléophas fell seriously ill. In the light of later evidence, it seems likely that he had tuberculosis. The man who now saved him was his newly adopted Parisian mentor, one of the great medical scientists of the day, Professor Jean-Noël Hallé (1754–1822). Achille-Cléophas had struck lucky once again. Hallé was the most influential and the most kindly mentor imaginable. In his qualifying dissertation of 1810, Achille-Cléophas paid tribute to him as the man whose teaching he valued the most. 'My gratitude to him is proportionate to both the knowledge I owe to him and to the intelligent care he lavished upon me [...] during a very serious illness.' Achille-Cléophas also gratefully incorporated Hallé's principles of hygiene into his dissertation.[14]

In the disdainfully competitive world of Parisian medicine, Hallé was the conspicuous and benevolent exception. His colleagues spoke well of him, far beyond the formal requirements of funeral oratory. 'The young doctors he gathered around him will never forget that he treated them with great respect and kindness, that he encouraged them in all their efforts, bestowing his patronage on men of talent and probity.'[15] Hallé's generous temperament also found expression in his dealing with his patients. He was, according to Cuvier's formal tribute, 'a man naturally kind, and his patients adored him. When all was lost, he knew how, by his drollery, to make the sufferer forget his troubles.'[16] A gifted, generous and energetic teacher, a man of many accomplishments with a legendary capacity for hard work, Hallé, now in his late forties, enjoyed a secure and prominent position at the heart of the Parisian medical and scientific world. An agile survivor of every recent change of regime, he served as personal physician to Napoleon, then to Charles X and to Louis XVIII.

Amongst his many achievements, Hallé was the creator of the discipline of medical hygiene, a discipline with an impressive future under

its later name, public health. Elaborating a theme familiar from the contemporary ideologue project for a science of man, Hallé explored the
medical implications of the materialist arguments for the unity of the
physical and the moral. The whole enterprise was not exclusively scientific. It had an explicit moral and political purpose, in harmony with the
radical national project of regeneration. According to Hallé, writing in
1792, a moment at which almost everything still seemed possible, 'it is
in the sphere of public hygiene that the enlightened physician becomes
the counsellor and the guide of the legislator.'[17]

It would survive beyond the revolutionary decade, this idea of the
social mission and the cultural authority of the enlightened physician. On
the other hand, to accomplish that mission was going to require an alliance
of professional interests so complex and so politically contentious that
Achille-Cléophas's generation would not live to see it. Achille-Cléophas
would one day be appointed as the first head of a regional health council.
However, as a physician who specialised in surgery, he remained loyal
to the narrower ideal of individual clinical competence. At a later date,
he would find himself in bitter conflict with his colleague, Hellis, who
practised a conservative statistical form of social medicine.

IT WAS PROBABLY THROUGH HALLÉ'S INFLUENCE that Achille-Cléophas,
as a medical student, came into contact with two of the foremost scientists of the day. The more memorable of the two was undoubtedly Baron
Alexander von Humboldt, the celebrated Prussian traveller and naturalist. In the eyes of his admiring contemporaries, Humboldt, now in his
mid-thirties, was the embodiment of the intellectual romance of science.
He had just returned from an ambitious voyage around South America,
and he was in Paris between August 1804 and the spring of 1805. There
he 'maintained a lively intercourse with the most eminent scholars of the
capital',[18] recruiting a wide circle of collaborators to assist in documenting
his discoveries. Hallé and Humboldt came together at this point. We can
see them, in a contemporary engraving, companionably dissecting frogs.[19]

At some point, during that winter of 1804–5, Achille-Cléophas was
delegated to give Humboldt a series of anatomy lessons. It was presumably
a mark of great favour, for the young medical student to be summoned,
however fleetingly, into this elite metropolitan circle of scientific gentlemen. Was he paid or did he do it for *la gloire*? In view of his temporary

student poverty, and his eventual conspicuous wealth, I incline to think that Achille-Cléophas was indeed paid.

Be that as it may, he evidently recalled the episode with some satisfaction. The fact that it is mentioned in the obituary pamphlet of 1847 suggests that Achille-Cléophas spoke of it to his colleagues many years later, confident that it would be taken as an informal mark of distinction. Predictably, this contact with Humboldt had no sequel. At the dissecting table, the Baron could happily learn from Achille-Cléophas; thereafter Humboldt strolled away into a world of conviviality, erudition and privilege that the capable youth from Nogent-sur-Seine could scarcely imagine. We can be fairly confident that Achille-Cléophas was *not* present in the audience at the Paris Institute on 7 December 1804 when Humboldt delivered to that eminent gathering a memoir describing his discovery of the decrease in intensity of the Earth's magnetic force from the poles to the equator.

After Humboldt, Achille-Cléophas disappears from the grand narrative of science, immersing himself in professional concerns of compelling local importance. In 1846, according to the probate inventory of his estate, there was no Humboldt in his library. The habit of unremunerative intellectual ambition evidently survived until around the moment of his mid-thirties; we shall see that Achille-Cléophas delivers a series of eleven observations and reports to the Rouen Academy in the five years between 1815 and 1820. Thereafter, he leaves few traces in the general archives of his profession. As will be clear, the Rouen Academy in those post-Restoration years was not the place for unbuttoned intellectual audacity of the Humboldt vintage.

More prosaically, though also worthy of recall, Achille-Cléophas worked as a demonstrator in the laboratory of the chemist Louis Jacques Thénard (1771–1856). He and Thénard and had much in common. Thénard was only seven years his senior; he had been to same school as Achille-Cléophas; he came from the same region, and from a family of modest tenant farmers. In 1802, at the age of twenty-five, Thénard had made his mark by synthesising cobalt blue, a pigment used in the production of luxury porcelain. To be working in Thénard's laboratory, at this point, was to find oneself in contact with youthful scientific genius of modest social origin.

Four volumes of Thénard were found in Achille-Cléophas's library. For any physician, chemistry was the key science. Achille-Cléophas's inaugural speech to the Rouen Academy in 1815, as it runs through the whole repertoire of the sciences, dwells at some length upon the utility of chemistry:

> What a truly immense fund of knowledge does chemistry offer to the physician! The nature and the properties, whether useful or harmful, of the different gases; the composition of the air, the qualities that make it suitable for animal respiration, the means of measuring its purity and of cleansing it when insalubrious, the procedures to combat the deleterious effects of putrid miasmas, the preparation of medicines of all kinds, the nature of poisons, animal, vegetable and mineral, their mode of operation, the most effective methods of controlling their harmful effects, the changes undergone by animal liquids and solids, under the influence of different diseases, the most effective measures to be taken to halt their progress and to alleviate the disorders which they have already produced; such are the important areas in which the physician can only attain an exact knowledge by the study of the principles of chemistry.[20]

In *Madame Bovary*, it is a measure of the mediocrity of the village pharmacist, Homais, that he makes a simple mistake over the chemical composition of methane. The fact that Charles Bovary, the village doctor, doesn't notice Homais's mistake is equally to *his* discredit. They are both incompetent.

Achille-Cléophas's professional competence was never in question. 'In medicine, mediocrity is a crime.' This was one of most resonant sayings. For three successive years, as a medical student, he won first prize in his section. Beyond the pleasant surge in self-esteem, these prizes meant that his fees were rescinded. Among his student cohort, Achille-Cléophas was conspicuously successful. At this point, his early biographer slips into the mildly grandiose idiom of the Homeric warrior-hero:

> He took part in all the competitive exams and, every time, emerged victorious from the struggle. His superiority was so well known to his adversaries that on several occasions (we have this fact from one of those adversaries who used to enjoy telling the story) he would sell to his friends, in advance, the books that were to be the victor's reward, and he took the money in advance of the results.[21]

For all his academic prowess, and for all his cherished connections with Humboldt and Thénard, Achille-Cléophas did not become a medical scientist. Like his blacksmith and veterinary ancestors, he worked with his hands, as a surgeon, as a superior artisan, immersed in the material world. Like Charles Bovary, Achille-Cléophas will 'thrust his hand down into damp beds, have his face splashed with warm-spurting blood, listen to many a death-rattle, examine the contents of chamber-pots, and unbutton plenty of grubby under-linen'.[22]

THOUGH ACHILLE-CLÉOPHAS WAS NOT conspicuously a man to take his ease, he somehow found time, as a student in Paris, to cultivate a circle that was distinctly not part of his enclosed primary medical world. He was a regular visitor to the salon of J.-B. Salgues, a man whom he liked and admired, formerly the director of the college in Sens, now a Parisian and a man of letters. In that salon there assembled 'the great men and the great trollops of the day'.[23] Only one name from that salon group has found its way into the record: the writer Népomucène Lemercier (1771–1840). Lemercier, then in his early thirties but once a child prodigy and latterly a fashionable poet and dramatist, was, at least until the year 1803, a member of Napoleon's inner circle. When Achille-Cléophas made the acquaintance of Lemercier he was working on an epic poem in six books, *L'Atlantiade*. This was a belated specimen of that hybrid genre of late eighteenth-century verse, the neo-classical science-poem. Essentially a periphrastic celebration of Newton and of the mathematical harmonies of the universe, its official subtitle was 'A Newtonian Theogeny'. Its joke-subtitle was 'The Loves of the Elements'.[24]

The salon was still a place for reading aloud from one's work in progress; we may thus picture Achille-Cléophas, more bemused than impressed, feeling somewhat constrained in this unfamiliar setting, listening to generous portions of *L'Atlantiade* declaimed by their author from manuscript. Aside from any awkward questions as to the merits of *L'Atlantiade*, it is worth observing that science and poetry had not yet parted company, in the public and professional discourse of this generation. Physicians could publish in verse and in prose, expecting to be taken equally seriously.

8

Conscription

Never had there been so many sleepless nights as in the time of that man; never had there been seen, hanging over the ramparts of the cities, such a nation of desolate mothers; never was there such a silence about those who spoke of death. And yet in all hearts never was there such joy, such life, such fanfares of war.

— ALFRED DE MUSSET, *The Confession of a Child of the Century* (1836)

WHEN ACHILLE-CLÉOPHAS TURNED TWENTY in November 1804, he became potentially liable for five years of military service in the armies of the Empire. After a decade of war against the assembled monarchies of Europe, France's administrative machinery for processing conscripts was now formidably effective. The annual levy for Achille-Cléophas's year would take place in September 1805. Potential conscripts drew numbers in a lottery. The lower your number, the stronger the chances that you would be included in the annual military levy. If Achille-Cléophas drew a low number, he would have to set about finding a way to avoid military service.

There were various ways to do this, not all of them legal. If you were poor, you might decide to go into hiding before they came for you. On the other hand, you could desert the colours, once you were in uniform. Many, in great despair, mutilated themselves cruelly, in order to be declared unfit for service. Teeth were pulled out, hernias induced, genitalia damaged by the application of corrosive fluids.[1]

If you had money, you had more choices. You could pay for someone to take your place. That was legal but, as the wars dragged on, it was ever more expensive. A replacement could cost the equivalent of ten years' income for a farm labourer. It was often cheaper to find an inconspicuously corrupt local official who could sell you a fraudulent certificate of exemption. The trade in fraudulent exemptions was splendidly lucrative. Municipal officials making sudden and conspicuous acquisitions of property were often summoned to give an account of their good fortune.[2]

On 4 July 1806, Achille-Cléophas attended an army medical examination in the town of Troyes, administrative centre for the Department of the Aube. The army doctor, one Captain Robert, certified that Achille-Cléophas, 'conscript from Year XIV', was henceforth exempt from military service, on the grounds that he was 'suffering from pulmonary phthisis'. The fee for the certificate was 65 francs, quite a substantial sum of money.[3]

Colloquially, Achille-Cléophas had consumption. *Phthisis* was the late eighteenth-century term for that large group of diseases that had yet to be differentiated. Tuberculosis was not isolated and named until the late 1830s. This certified fact, whether true or false, was going to make all the difference to the future course of his life. It may well have been true. At the very least, it was not improbable. Achille-Cléophas was an underfed medical student, working to the very limits of his energies, living in damp urban conditions, routinely exposed to sources of infection and to the generally polluted air of the great city. He had also been seriously and authentically ill during his first winter in the capital.

On the other hand, the exemption may have been false. Several features of his subsequent history suggest that this was the case. Achille-Cléophas was going to survive a further forty years, without any obvious history of ill health, apart from the last years of his life. He not only survived, but also worked strenuously and consistently in a demanding position, as well as raising three children, none of whom were infected. The evidence suggests an exceptionally strong constitution.

If it was false, how might the deception have been accomplished? As the son of a man fairly recently acquitted of fraud and unpatriotic utterances, Achille-Cléophas was likely to be cautious in his dealings with the finely engineered Napoleonic state apparatus. It might be risky and expensive to try to bribe either the military doctor or one of the many local officials responsible for the paperwork behind the conscription process. Better to call upon one's influential superiors and sound them out. Such manoeuvres to avoid conscription were not unknown in medical circles. The whole business could be dealt with off the record. No money need change hands and there would be nothing in writing. It was a professional favour, a reward for exceptional merit, a discreet vote of confidence in one's abilities. We don't know for sure who may have acted on his behalf to secure the exemption. In one plausible version of the story, it was Achille-Cléophas's immediate superior, Dupuytren, and the exemption was the reward for agreeing to depart from Paris.

Over and above any personal reluctance to wear uniform, the army medical corps was no place for an enlightened physician in 1806. Napoleon disliked men who professed their belief in observation, experiment and the power of the individual mind. The humanitarian medical ethos was regarded as an encumbrance. Military strategy and administrative efficiency were the sole imperatives of the hour. Talented individual physicians, however courageous and conscientious, would find themselves frustrated in their efforts by a policy that amounted to simply abandoning the wounded on the battlefield.[4]

In terms of his rapid professional advancement, exemption from military service was the best thing that could happen to Achille-Cléophas. Obviously, the workings of conscription would reduce the competition, and the exemption would allow him to concentrate on the next step, the writing of the required dissertation. At this turning point in his career, Achille-Cléophas was helped on his way by the formidable machinery of medical patronage, now restored to working order.[5]

It was supremely fortunate that the dean of the Paris Health School, Michel Augustin Thouret (1748–1810), held Achille-Cléophas in high regard. In the late summer of 1806, learning of a vacancy for an anatomy demonstrator at the Hôtel-Dieu in Rouen, Thouret decided to recommend Achille-Cléophas for the post. Thouret then instructed a younger colleague, one Guillaume Dupuytren, assistant chief surgeon at the Hôtel-Dieu in Paris, to write the letter of recommendation. These indirect tactics may have been devised to avoid any appearance of nepotism, given that the chief surgeon in Rouen was Thouret's brother-in-law. Whatever the reason, Dupuytren was now the active party in securing Achille-Cléophas's appointment to the position in Rouen.

Dupuytren's letter has survived in the regional archives. It offers a fascinating official portrait of Achille-Cléophas at the end of his Parisian medical apprenticeship. Dupuytren talks him up in the strongest terms. He tells his Rouen colleague that Achille-Cléophas will be a great asset, solid in character as well as exceptionally talented. He is a young man who has inspired great hopes among his senior colleagues in Paris.

> I must tell you that Monsieur Flaubert has been successful in the internal competition for positions in the Paris hospitals and that for the last two years he has carried out these duties in the most honourable fashion; that he has equally been entered for the examinations for the École Pratique and that he has obtained the first prize in every class, an achievement which has entitled him to have his fees rescinded, an honour which the school has introduced for the first time; finally […] this year he has won the Institute's first prize for anatomy and physiology. This, dear sir, is the demonstrator I am sending to you; I shall add […] that for several years he has been one of my students and one of my particular friends and that I shall be infinitely grateful to you for all that you care to do for his instruction and his advancement, as well as for the accommodation which such a well-brought-up young man will need.[6]

Achille-Cléophas was duly appointed as the demonstrator in anatomy at the Hôtel-Dieu in Rouen. As such, he would now be responsible for giving a series of public anatomy lessons, as well as for working in the recently founded Rouen School of Artificial Anatomy, collaborating in the making of life-size three-dimensional wax replicas of dissected human body parts. To be appointed to this position was a consecration of the intellectual excellence that Achille-Cléophas had pursued so tirelessly for so many years. He could expect to remain in Rouen for a year or two and then move on to even greater things. To Paris perhaps, where the very best of the profession were assembled in valiant mutual emulation.

Looking back upon this wonderfully decisive moment in his professional life, Achille-Cléophas became convinced that Dupuytren's motives in supporting him were, to say the least, questionable. His other mentors, Salgues, Hallé and Thouret, each inspired an uncomplicated gratitude. Dupuytren, on the other hand, was more like an older brother who pushes the younger around, saying that it is because he knows best. This singularly negative moral fact only became clear to Achille-Cléophas in later years when he discovered, through the workings of professional gossip, how very unpleasant a character the great Dupuytren was known to be.[7]

For all his talent, Dupuytren was indeed notoriously vindictive towards his professional rivals. He was, in the judgement of one of his colleagues, the first of surgeons and the least of men. His pupils remembered him 'striding along the corridors like a God on Earth, pontificating and oblivious', awkward, insolent and aggressive, not averse to intrigue or to plagiarism, bullying his patients who were terrified in his presence.[8] Knowing some version of all this, in later years Achille-Cléophas detected a plot by Dupuytren to banish him to the provinces, to get him out of the way for fear that he might one day become a threat to Dupuytren's supposedly precarious pre-eminence. Achille-Cléophas evidently shared these ugly suspicions with his colleagues, for the story of Dupuytren's treachery makes its way, substantially, into the obituary memoir that Védie published in the year after his death.

Here it is, from that source, the 'authorised version' of Dupuytren's turpitude:

> This egotism, which kept him constantly alert, must have led him to suspect what Flaubert might one day become. He conceived a way to get rid of him. Flaubert's poor state of health supplied a convenient pretext: twisting this circumstance to his selfish advantage, Dupuytren earnestly advised his pupil to leave Paris and move to Normandy. There was not enough money to cover the essential expenses; he found the sum required and lent the young man six hundred francs to cover the cost of the journey and the other expenses of moving; and so the young man set out, with few possessions, but a rich future ahead of him.[9]

Whether or not the allegation is true, this fixed belief, evidently shared with colleagues, that he was tricked into leaving Paris, becomes in itself a curious psychological fact about Achille-Cléophas. Stories of his ferocious temper point in the same direction: this was a man who gave everything to his profession and yet he struggled with demons that gathered in the dark to mock him as a failure.

9

A Century of Marvels

Receive my modest tribute, you in whom we all admire that imperturbable sang-froid, so vital to the success of a surgical operation, that special skill, that quality of determination that is so rapidly superseded by a gentle feeling of pity, that scrupulous care to minimise pain, in a word that happy combination of all the qualities that make an excellent surgeon.

— D.M. VIGNÉ, *Obituary for a Surgeon* (1818)

O N 27 NOVEMBER 1806, Achille-Cléophas arrived in Rouen, after a three-day journey in the *diligence*, the fast public stagecoach. He was just twenty-two. Quite fortuitously, we know what he looked like from the sketchy physical details recorded on his certificate of exemption from military service. He was five feet nine inches tall, with brown eyes, an oval-shaped face, a long nose and a small chin.

To a young man anticipating an unaccustomed burden in his wallet, a young man just released from prolonged years of student poverty, the city of Rouen might wear, at least on that first day, the aspect of a feast spread out before him. He might now begin to acquire a taste for the civilised pleasures, *les menus plaisirs*, appropriate to his new status. The latest books, a sober wardrobe of well-made clothes, several pairs of not purely sensible shoes, an evening's frivolous entertainment: for the first time, in a life so single-minded, these things all lay within reach.

Here is Vallée frères, the local bookshop, where he can buy, for twenty-five francs, the new translation of Adam Smith's *Wealth of Nations*, in five octavo volumes.[1] In a lighter vein, he might browse through the pages of the *Letter on the Perils of Onanism*, an edifying work 'useful for fathers and teachers'.[2] Rouen's Théâtre des Arts is offering *Le Caravane de Caire*, a grand opera on a fashionable oriental-imperial theme.[3] At the other end of the cultural marketplace, the Equestrian Amphitheatre is playing *Don Quixote*, billed as a burlesque pantomime in two acts, with battles and gymnastic interludes, featuring Monsieur Forioso's elder sister dancing upon the tightrope.[4]

But these are mere frivolities. The official mood of the hour is caught in the closing words of the local newspaper announcement for *The Dream*, a topical-patriotic Christmas miscellany that will be playing throughout December at the Théâtre des Arts.

> The high deeds that continue to distinguish the genius of the emperor and the courage of his great and valiant army offer to the imagination such wonders that we are inclined to think we are dreaming when we read the bulletins which set out each glorious circumstance, were it not for the fact that we are in the century of marvels, quite accustomed to seeing ever new and ever more extraordinary things brought about.[5]

The century of marvels, defined principally by Napoleon's current exploits, was now in its sixth wonderful year. The week before Achille-Cléophas arrived in Rouen, Napoleon had arrived in Berlin and set about issuing proclamations. The emperor's victory bulletin was printed on the front page of the *Journal de Rouen*. On the inside page there was a 'Patriotic Ode on the Prussian War' in eight stanzas.[6] According to instructions from Paris, the latest imperial victory was to be celebrated in the nation's churches, 'in gratitude to the Supreme Being who so visibly guides and protects the invincible armies of His Imperial Majesty'.[7]

IN THE WINTER OF 1806 the fashionable local patriot, with one eye on the Supreme Being and the other on the value of his investments, can be observed wearing a long-tailed, white-buttoned version of the Napoleonic greatcoat. In Rouen the linen merchants are selling great quantities of an elaborately festooned lace *jabot*.[8] In Les Halles, Rouen's great seventeenth-century Cloth Hall, there is brisk trading in fabrics whose very names evoke a lost world of precise sartorial nuance: *siamoise*, white thread and worsted, fustian, drill and check. These are the city's commercial speciality, *la fabrique rouennaise*, plain everyday fabrics for the masses, the no-nonsense stuff of a peasant woman's skirt, the bright colours of a regimental uniform.

The local cotton industry took off in the first decade of this century of marvels. By the year 1806, Rouen was a very good place to make money. Let us follow the story of the making of one particular cotton millionaire, Pierre-Jean Le Verdier. A man of the same generation as Achille-Cléophas, Le Verdier was the son of a labourer from a village on the road to Dieppe. He arrived in Rouen in 1800, the year that the first six-horse-power steam engine was installed in a local cotton-spinning mill. At this time, in this place, it was still relatively easy to set up with only modest capital. Local conditions were favourable. *La fabrique rouennaise* was about to take off. Waterpower was cheap and abundant, thanks to the geology of the local river basin. Labour was also cheap and abundant, with a local population accustomed to textile work. Convent and monastery buildings, recently sequestered from the church, converted nicely to industrial uses. The financial structure of the industry allowed for many modest proto-industrial units of production to thrive alongside the big beasts. One could start somewhere near the bottom of the pile and then rise to a great height.[9]

By 1807, after only seven years, Le Verdier had set up in business on his own. On the back of an advantageous marriage, he went into partnership with a big Parisian company and soon bought out their Rouen branch. He was no longer a primary producer. He supplied raw materials, he sold the finished product, he rented out a dye-works and he lent money to other manufacturers. As he prospered, he moved into real estate, buying farms and land. The crowning moment came in 1840 when Le Verdier bought the chateau in his native village of Belmesnil and became mayor. He left a fortune of two million francs to his nine children; Pierre, the eldest, inherited the chateau and promptly married into the aristocracy.[10]

It was a characteristic progression, from workshop to factory to chateau, with an aristocratic marriage in the next generation. Achille-Cléophas himself will soon enact his own version of that same story of social advancement. He will marry up, make money, buy land and live eventually in a very large country house that will be the equal of any chateau. His best friend will be a liberal industrialist, a man on the make, like himself. Rouen is not Paris, but it will prove immensely congenial and Achille-Cléophas will remain here for forty years.

THE CITY STANDS ON A WIDE BEND of the river Seine, halfway between Paris and the ocean. The river is tidal here. You can smell the salt, like a bright pleasant memory of the open sea. In 1806 that smell is lost in among the thick, damp folds of the ubiquitous, excremental, nineteenth-century urban stench. Wooden sailing ships, a thousand ships every year, are moored at the busy quayside. What currents of money must flow, swift and exhilarating, into the coffers of these citizens. The imposing remains of city walls, a multitude of elegant church spires, the rows of solidly handsome stone-built townhouses: they all testify to five centuries of prosperity and contentment. The merchants and the manufacturers of Rouen draw excellent profits from cheap textiles, mass-produced pottery and the regional cider market. Plain-living, money-loving men, they share a mild disdain for all the capricious, sword-carrying, silk-stockinged, white-wigged creatures of the recent past.

Rouen is a city of commerce. Dedicated to the pursuit of material interests, its citizens are notoriously indifferent to both religion and politics. This aspect of the local culture will suit the new arrival, though it troubles the government of the day. Religious indifference was measured by the numbers attending Easter mass. In 1805, a report from the local prefect stated that only one in four of the women and one in fifty of the men took communion. None of those men held any public office in the city. The Napoleonic elite, many of them owners of sequestered church property, largely ignored spiritual matters. Factory owners and workers showed their scorn for religion by working on Sundays.[11]

Ever since 1790 there had been no bishop in the city of Rouen. Church land and church buildings had been sequestered and put to new and profane uses. When bishops were restored in 1802, the new incumbent, one Étienne-Hubert de Cambacérès, came from a family belonging to the legal nobility of the Ancien Régime. He and his older brother, an eminent jurist, had supported the Revolution, though they had opposed the execution of the king. Both brothers were now in high favour with Napoleon. The new bishop, a proverbial safe pair of hands, knew that he had best play his cards carefully with these godless locals. Not too many combative religious processions. No gratuitous threats of damnation against freemasons and radicals. One worked best with the ladies, coaxing them into public acts of charity.

ACHILLE-CLÉOPHAS ENDS HIS JOURNEY at the Hôtel-Dieu de Rouen. A refuge for the indigent sick, the Hôtel-Dieu was an enduring, imposing emblem of the church's social mission. Then as now, it was a place of formal splendour. As big as a palace, it's a great geometrical complex of neo-classical public buildings that still breathes an austere French grandeur. Built in several stages between the years 1650 and 1770, the Hôtel-Dieu had been a prison, a warehouse and a barracks, before it became a hospital. The last doctor left the building in 1962. Expensively renovated in the 1990s, the Hôtel-Dieu now serves as the regional *préfecture*, a labyrinthine urban chateau housing the elegant and genial administrative elite of the day. Arriving early in the winter of 1806, Achille-Cléophas was to spend the next forty years of his working life in this building. He would need an informed understanding of its history, its purpose and its institutional form.

As a large walled city, huddled around a busy port, Rouen had long been the perfect place to catch the plague. Smallpox, dysentery, scarlet fever, raw sewage and horse-dung were the ingredients in this witches' brew of urban mortality. The charitable citizens of Rouen had thus decreed, long ago, that a religious hospital, the Hôtel-Dieu, was to be built in the shadow of their great cathedral. There, in the Hôtel-Dieu, where all human misery was gathered in, you might pray to St Roch for a miracle and prepare your soul for the quiet of the afterlife. As the city grew so the dangers of contagion increased and it became evident that something more modern, more sensibly remote was required. In July 1758 the sick were lifted, coaxed and bullied from their beds in the old Hôtel-Dieu. Singing psalms, carrying crosses and candles, they were carted across the city in a symbolically edifying procession and shown to their new quarters, a splendid neo-classical edifice, situated on open ground just beyond the city walls.

The sick now found themselves, on that eighteenth-century July day, installed in cavernous rooms with the names of saints: Louis, Madeleine, Sebastian, Marguerite and Ambroise. Bright spacious rooms, they were heated by massive cast-iron stoves. Here in these church-sized spaces the sick were crowded together, five in each enormous bed. Their mattresses, irregularly stuffed with fresh straw, gave off a nostalgic smell of summer fields. Augustinian nuns dressed in white robes, black veils and black capes decorated with the large scarlet cross of Malta watched over the godly and the ungodly alike. They brewed rich herbal potions in the giant vats of the *tisanerie*; they recited Latin prayers over the dying; they sewed together the rough sacks in which the plague-corpses were hurriedly laid to rest. Expelled from their functions in 1790 along with the rest of the more refractory clergy, the nuns had returned in 1802. In their baggage they brought with them a cherished life-size polychrome wooden statue of St Agatha, her martyred breasts displayed bleeding on a large dish, for all the world like an underdone Sunday roast. One wonders, compassionately, what thoughts St Agatha prompted in the minds of female patients arriving for surgery.

Achille-Cléophas had no need to write any description of this institution in which he spent so many years of his life. However, in 1826, one of his colleagues, Dr Hellis, published the following brief account of the workings of the Hôtel-Dieu.

> The Hôtel-Dieu is dedicated to the treatment of curable conditions both chronic and acute, both inpatients and outpatients. Each year nearly four thousand patients are admitted, along with six or seven hundred soldiers or sailors. All patients are housed in separate beds in spacious rooms, according to the type and the severity of their illness. The majority are medical patients; around one third of the total are treated on the surgical wards, by Monsieur Flaubert and Monsieur Leudet, his deputy, men worthy of the brilliant tradition that comes down from Lecat. One ward is set aside for the soldiers, one for pregnant women in labour. The latter ward is set up for the instruction of student midwives, directed by the senior midwife, subject to inspection by the medical and the surgical directors. In addition there is a ward specifically for children under the age of five, and several rooms for the elderly. Separate from the patients housed in the main building, there are three or four hundred contagious patients […]. Free consultations are available every day to the indigent, for the instruction of the medical students, consisting of four interns and twenty externs, all exclusively employed in the surgical division.
>
> The pharmacy, unsurpassed of its kind, apart from supplying the medicines used on the premises, also supplies whatever has been prescribed by the physicians of the twelve local charities.[12]

The pharmacy, one of the great and necessary spaces of the medical world, is worth exploring in more detail. Traditionally, the nuns run the pharmacy. They are known to sell remedies in town and they have no formal training. On both accounts, they are often in conflict with the qualified pharmacists. In 1806, the pharmacy stands opposite the main entrance gate, on the ground floor, to the right of the courtyard, next to the kitchens and the laundry. It takes the form of a suite of rooms; in the *tisanerie* they process the raw materials; in the dispensary they mix the potions; in the storeroom they keep the finished product. There is a herb garden just at the back, with a specially constructed water tank.

The *tisanerie* is large rectangular space with walls of immense thickness. It is a bare-brick cave with heavy vaulting and deeply recessed windows, designed to create great pools of perpetual shadow. To the more imaginative visitor, the *tisanerie* looks like an alchemist's secret workshop. There is a monumental central stove with an array of huge copper alembics, all their curves gleaming. Your guide points out that the alembic is in three parts. There is the gourd-shaped lower vessel. That is called the *cucurbit*. Then there is the tapering *headpiece* and then the *worm*, the tall condensing coil that distils the infusions of medicinal herbs.

All around there are shelves crowded with implements: wooden presses, copper pans, cauldrons, kettles, retorts, balloon flasks, ewers and glazed jugs. There is a splendid cold-water tap shaped like a swan's neck. There are giant mortars, made of iron, bronze or marble, for grinding and mixing. The pestle is far too big to work by hand. It has to be dropped into an iron ring mounted on the wall. For grinding toxic ingredients, you must put a soft leather cover over the mortar, so as not to inhale the dust.

Next door to the *tisanerie* is the dispensary, a place of imposing beauty and order. The walls are covered from floor to ceiling with wooden panels, all painted grey. In the centre of the room there sits a large workbench, elaborately fitted out, like some giant child's toy, with shelves and drawers, cupboards and pigeonholes. Dried herbs are kept below. Medicinal powders are stored up above in little boxes. On the workbench, for weighing out the ingredients, there are brass scales in all different sizes. Neatly arrayed, each in its cupboard or on its shelf, there are intimidating enema syringes, silver feeding bottles, pill compresses, boxes of weights and leather bags for spices.

In pride of place, here are the so-called sovereign remedies. They are stored in sumptuously decorated vessels, all elegantly labelled. *Theriac*, a great panacea, is a confection of opium and viper meat. *Orvietan* is a confection of wine, dissolved honey and toxic herbs. *Confection of Hyacinth* is made from yellow zircon. It is for palpitation of the heart.

Even for ordinary ingredients, there is a range of exotic vessels. The *Chevrette* is a pear-shaped jug with a spout like a little horn for syrups and oils. The *Albarello* is a cylindrical majolica jar with a concave waist, used for balms, ointments, waxes, electuaries and opiates. It is sealed with a piece of parchment or leather, tied round with a piece of cord. The *Monster* is a large oval jar on a pedestal. As well as its exuberant floral decoration, the *Monster* has two handles in the form of serpents entwined, an ornate cover and a cartouche inscribed with the mysterious Latin name of the remedy within. Polychrome porcelain vessels have recently replaced the old earthenware kind. They come with a symbolic decoration depicting the three kingdoms of nature: animal, vegetable and mineral. That is the slightly elusive meaning the image of the palm tree growing on rocky ground with a serpent wrapped around the trunk.[13]

From the month of his arrival in Rouen, Achille-Cléophas's career seemed to follow a smoothly ascending curve. As the demonstrator attached to the School of Anatomy and Medicine he was apprenticed to an illustrious new master, Jean-Baptiste Laumonier. This was the man he would need to impress. As it turned out, he would indeed do so, with conspicuous success.

Laumonier, now in his mid-fifties, had been chief surgeon at the Hôtel-Dieu de Rouen for the past twenty years. Trained in Paris, he had then worked in a military hospital in the northeast before coming to Rouen in 1784. There, within three years, Laumonier married into the local elite. His wife, *née* Thouret, had brothers in high places, medical, legal and political. Michel Thouret was the first director of the Health School in Paris. Jacques Thouret was a prominent local lawyer, eventually elected as deputy for Rouen in the National Assembly. Like his brother-in-law Jacques, the Laumonier of the early 1790s initially welcomed the Revolution, even though it cost him his income from the *octroi*, the toll charged on merchandise entering the town. In 1792 Laumonier was elected as director of the Rouen Academy of Arts and Sciences. This soon became a dangerous place to be, at the heart of the civic culture of the day. Laumonier was about to be conscripted, against his own inclinations, into the politics of the day. Unlike his eminent brother-in-law, executed in the purge of the Girondins in 1794, Laumonier survived, though not unscathed.

By the year 1806, most persons of any importance had their individual survival story, crafted and polished. Laumonier's story was exceptionally instructive, a piece of valuable political wisdom, to be imparted to one's receptive younger colleagues as a lesson in the perils of political enthusiasm. I suggest that Laumonier's story, as it eventually emerged, confirmed Achille-Cléophas in his cautious, pragmatic, elite liberalism. As with any generation entangled in a traumatic collective history, the double task of remembering and forgetting would be carried forward, little by little, year after year, all through life.

There were two splendidly bizarre items in Laumonier's collection of medical curiosities: the shrunken, severed heads of Citizens François Bordier and Thomas-Charles Jourdain. Scientifically preserved according to a secret process devised by Laumonier, these two heads still sit side by side in a display cabinet in Rouen's Museum of the History of Medicine. These are not skulls, the soothingly blank relics of mortality. These are human heads, the very seat of individual identity. Their faces are expressive and more or less intact. The skin covering the face is a leathery, creamy brown, with a few darker patches. The hair and the teeth, the lips, the noses and the ears are all present and correct. Their two pairs of bright blue glass eyes meet the gaze of posterity with a disconcerting fixity.

In Rouen in 1806, everyone of a certain age knew the story of the two severed heads. When I visited the museum, in the last decade of the twentieth century, venerable anti-Jacobin jokes on the subject of these two severed heads were still circulating. 'That's Bordier and Jourdain', said my guide. 'They made the revolution too soon. Jumped the gun.' Decapitated and mockingly demonised, Bordier and Jourdain had once, for a few weeks, been men to reckon with. In the month of August 1789, they were the leaders of a violent popular insurrection that turned the city upside down. For a few memorable days, the local merchant elite lost the political control it would otherwise maintain, more or less, all through the years of the Revolution.[14]

The summer of 1789 was a time of ecstatic popular violence, known to history as the Great Fear. The month of July, just before the grain harvest, was always the hungriest time of the year. This particular July was explosive. Collective emotion took the form of food riots and machine breaking. The soldiers fraternised with crowds they had been sent to disperse. Royal officials fled for their lives. Rouen thought it had escaped the worst of the Great Fear, but by early August the administration was losing control of the city.

The hostile official narrative, even though compiled some fifty years after the event, is still pulsing with anxiety. At the centre of the action was Thomas Jourdain, a local lawyer. He rose to sudden intoxicating political power on the streets of Rouen, at the head of a small army of young men. They were the dregs, *hommes sans aveu*, masterless men.[15] A mix of local workers and soldiers who had deserted from the Navarre regiment, the hungry, angry crowd regarded Jourdain, literate and bourgeois, as their oracle. He used his power to 'work them up to mischief of all kinds'. He even had the colonel of the local volunteers under his thumb. Jourdain was soon joined at the head of the crowd by one Bordier, a comic actor of genius. Bordier was famous on several counts: for playing the part of Harlequin on the Parisian stage, for his active role in the storming of the Bastille and not least for his notorious gambling debts. Actors, previously despised, were now to be acknowledged as active citizens. After all, they had the essential performance skills for the new revolutionary theatre of street-corner eloquence: a trained memory, strong clear diction, experience of improvisation and an easy way with a crowd. The actor and the lawyer, together they were a formidable and perverse alliance of discursive talents.

Signs of serious unrest appeared in the first week of August. The city fathers were caught off-guard. One morning they were faced with anonymous handwritten posters calling for the death of four of the most powerful local officials, the *intendant*, the president of the parliament and two of the chief magistrates. The new voice of the people was casual and peremptory: 'There are four heads that must be struck off […] Otherwise we are lost. If you don't do it, you will be thought a nation of cowards'. Accordingly, on the night of 3 August, a 'horde of malcontents' gathered outside the intendant's townhouse, calling for his death. The local volunteers, the *garde bourgeoise*, melted away. It was the classic crisis of authority. When the soldiers in the street defect or fraternise, then the civil servants at their desks begin to make a list of documents that must be destroyed. The Rouen crowd were shouting 'Death to the hoarders! Death to Maussion! We want his head on a pike!' They broke into the house and they set to work, gleefully wrecking the opulent interior.

Maussion, the intendant, had already left, walking through the crowd, disguised as one of his own lackeys. The crowd broke into the cellars, drank the best wine and fell asleep. There is much emphasis on this scene in the official written account. The more sober remnant, led by Jourdain, pillaged the neighbouring convent, then the tax office, then the *hotel de ville*, 'eyes blazing', muttering threats and insults. When they discovered that the intendant had fled the town, they smashed the tollgates. Then they lit an immense bonfire on the old market square. Furniture, clothes, papers and kitchen utensils were all thrown into the flames. Carriages were dragged out of courtyards and pushed into the river. The soldiers looked on without firing a shot.

Next morning, the streets were quiet. After their improvised carnivalesque triumph, the crowd was wondering what to do next. In that silence, a bourgeois militia formed up and arrested Bordier the actor. Next day, led by Jourdain, the crowd forced the release of Bordier. It took several days to restore military discipline. The crowd dissolved. Deserters and mutineers were weeded out, hunted down and locked up. Jourdain was arrested and imprisoned. Bordier fled the city. The militia pursued him halfway to Paris and arrested him in a small village where, predictably, he was inciting a riot.

Magistrates were soon back at work, sentencing the rioters. To advertise the restoration of the rule of law, a double gallows had been set up, in a prominent public place, down by the river, on the quai de Paris. A large and threateningly sympathetic crowd assembled there to witness the double execution of Bordier and Jourdain. To deter any active popular protest, a loaded cannon had been put in place near the gallows, facing outwards.

The public hanging ought to have been the end of the story of Bordier and Jourdain. However, the crisis of authority was not yet over. Laumonier himself was about to enter the scene, with exceptionally unpleasant consequences. At the site of the hanging, two medical students, acting on Laumonier's instructions, removed the heads from the fresh corpses of Bordier and Jourdain. They then conveyed them to Laumonier, for *processing*. In itself, this was nothing unusual. Fresh, healthy corpses from executions were routinely conveyed to medical schools for dissection. But these were no ordinary corpses. They were highly charged political artefacts, the focus of popular anger. It was prudent to remove and preserve the heads, the identifying portion, so that these potent symbols of insurrection and its nemesis could remain in the possession of the legitimate authorities. In this decade, anatomists were often conscripted, willing or not, into the political process. They had such useful practical skills, managing the copious body parts generated by the twists and turns of the Revolution.

The two severed heads were labelled and put away under medical custody, and there they remained for several years. Then, in the autumn of 1793, as the Revolution entered its most radical phase, the city administration of Rouen decreed, under great pressure from Paris, that Bordier and Jourdain were now to be rehabilitated as 'martyrs of liberty'. Religious ritual, though recently proscribed, was easily turned, easily rewritten to serve a worthy secular purpose. Accordingly, in November 1793, there unfolded in Rouen an elaborate public ceremony of rehabilitation, 'as odious as it was ridiculous'. An altar appeared on the quai de Paris where the executions had taken place. The two severed heads were taken out of storage, fitted with red liberty bonnets and placed on the altar, along with flowers, an inscription in letters of gold and a surgeon's guarantee that these were indeed the very heads. Then came a long procession of citizens in identical liberty bonnets. There were deputies, the local Société populaire, local actors, the administration, the judiciary, a troop of girls all in white with tricolour belts and garlands of roses. Bordier and Jourdain were acclaimed. It was declared that the city would bear the cost of educating their children. Their widows would receive pensions. The quai de Paris would be renamed after them. Laumonier made a pious speech in praise of their bravery. Hymns to liberty were sung and the procession made its way to the Temple of Reason, formerly the cathedral, 'seat of lies, now the seat of truth'.

Less than two years later, by February 1795, the political culture had come full circle. The virtuous crimes of 1793 had now in their turn to be cleansed. Laumonier was denounced as a terrorist for his part in the rehabilitation ceremony. He wrote a memoir in self-defence and was duly pardoned.[16] The rehabilitation of Bordier and Jourdain was revoked. Their heads were returned to the keeping of medical science, where they still reside.

Aside from his more recent political troubles, Laumonier enjoyed a great reputation as a teacher of anatomy. He was a gifted amateur artist with an interest in natural philosophy. His speciality was that wonderfully repulsive late eighteenth-century artefact, the *cerisculpture*, the life-size, three-dimensional, brightly coloured wax effigy of the half-dissected human form. In May 1806, the year of Achille-Cléophas's arrival, Laumonier had been appointed director of the newly established Rouen School of Artificial Anatomy. He and his assistants were commissioned to construct anatomical models for the medical schools, for the Museum of Natural History and for all the main hospitals. In the service of this laudable project, Laumonier drew in the best medical students from all over France, though they generally stayed in Rouen for only a year or two before moving on to higher things.

The respectful official view of Laumonier's wax models is expressed in the following tribute that appeared just after his death in the local daily newspaper, *Le Journal de Rouen*:

> Inspired by the desire to render less repulsive a branch of knowledge that entails certain dangers for the practitioner, and to present in fixed and invariable form the results of his researches and of his long and laborious dissections, he established, after unbelievable work, infinite care and attention, a laboratory of artificial anatomy, in which the wax took shape beneath his hand, depicting in fine detail all the various forms that nature displays. Endowed with copious incidental knowledge as well as an elegant and discriminating taste, he had the skill to veil the hideously repulsive side of anatomical dissection, whilst yet preserving the exact truth of the phenomena he sought to portray.[17]

Achille-Cléophas privately regarded Laumonier's famous wax figures as a ridiculous waste of time. In his view, they had nothing to do with real anatomy, as it ought to be taught. One day it would be safe to vent his scorn, but for the moment he had to play his cards carefully. Laumonier, though indolent and old-fashioned, was nonetheless a man of some influence. He had friends in high places and his wife's relatives were prominent in Parisian politics. Laumonier also had an adopted daughter, a sad-eyed, dark-haired girl of thirteen called Caroline Fleuriot, an orphan and an heiress. Her presence would eventually become Dr Flaubert's principal reason for staying in Rouen.

10

Compassionate Knowledge

The human body is one of the most beautiful machines to leave the hands of the Creator. Self-knowledge assumes knowledge of the body, and knowledge of the body assumes knowledge of such a prodigious constellation of causes and effects that it must lead directly to the notion of an intelligence both wise and omnipotent.

— *Encyclopédie, ou dictionnaire raisonné des sciences, des arts et des métiers* (1751)

IT WAS EVIDENT to his colleagues that Laumonier was languishing. The man was feeling his way towards retirement. His health was weakening. On a bad day, he seemed mildly confused, as if he had suffered a minor stroke.[1] This persistent and ill-concealed infirmity of one's professional overlord made for a delicate situation. Tact was required. Laumonier was still only in his fifties. He had just been given a new fiefdom and he was not about to retire.

Before too long, Achille-Cléophas observed that there was no proper medical instruction available at the Hôtel-Dieu. Eagerly focused on his pet project of *cerisculpture*, Laumonier had neglected the teaching side of things for some years. Achille-Cléophas promptly 'set up a school on his own and taught anatomy without charging, on his own initiative, driven by the need to share the light of his generous and sympathetic mind with others'.[2] Results were excellent and he soon established an independent reputation for himself as an inspiring teacher.

In 1808, discreetly circumventing his increasingly incompetent superior, Achille-Cléophas gave a series of lectures entitled Studies in Physiology (a transcript of which is held in the library of the National Academy of Medicine in Paris). It was a virtuoso performance from a man of twenty-three. Achille-Cléophas draws upon vivid examples from across the whole of the natural world and gives his voice to the intense intellectual excitement of the new science. At this point in the history of the discipline, physiology was experimental, speculative and proleptic. Lecturing on physiology was, for these reasons, the perfect arena in which a young man might advertise his intimacy with the new.

Preserved in manuscript, in the form of comprehensive notes taken by a diligent student, the lectures are impressive, both for their confident lucidity and for their range of intellectual reference. In view of their ambition and substance, it is surprising that Achille-Cléophas made no attempt to publish them. The fact that he did not publish suggests that he was perhaps working in isolation, with neither the stimulus of emulation nor the nourishment of general scientific conversation in his immediate context. Without parading his omniscience, Achille-Cléophas draws together the many strands of his own recent initiation. As one might expect, the name of Bichat occurs prominently, five times in the course of the text. Buffon is also mentioned, with distinct affection. Richerand is the only other named contemporary. Natural philosophy has come of age and is no longer to be subject to religious authority.

The measured gesture of indifference comes out within the first minutes of the first lecture.

> This word *nature* has been given several meanings. Thus it means either the whole array of beings in the universe, or it may mean the creator of this same universe, or it may mean the result of the laws to which these beings are subject.[3]

In his opening remarks, Achille-Cléophas alternates between different versions of the materialist conception of the organic life:

> In inert bodies composed of molecules linked to each other by aggregation or of forms superimposed one upon the other. Among the vegetables and the animals, we discover tissues of various types, areolar, fibrillary, vascular, laminar, all intersecting, mingling together in every possible way, forming membranes and ducts.[4]

Growth, in inert bodies, takes place through super-position. In living bodies it takes place by a mutual receptiveness.[5]

Just as the conjunction of the organs forms the system so that conjunction of all the systems forms the individual which is nothing more than a complicated machine made up of a large number of gearwheels each of which plays its part in the conservation of the whole.[6]

He makes only one isolated reference to the existence of the supernatural. It comes in the course of a modest thought experiment that harks back to a late eighteenth-century argument for materialism. Mentioning God, even in a perfunctory way, remained a sensibly pious precaution, to avoid being vilified as an atheist. 'Imagine', says Achille-Cléophas,

the existence of a being that is continually aware of what is visible to him without his being able to avoid it; continually aware of what might be useful to him without his being able to grasp it. The idea is absurd, and it does not accord with the grandeur and the bounty of a creator God.[7]

Cuvier is the name behind several excursions into the recent discipline of comparative anatomy:

The man to whom the study of anatomy and especially the study of comparative anatomy has become familiar, when he sees an organ taken from the body of an animal he will be able to deduce therefrom the structure of all those organs which composed that individual and he will be able to describe the modifications which they have undergone.[8]

In the case of a carnivore, the senses of sight, hearing, taste and smell will be more highly developed; the carnivore needs to move suddenly and rapidly to secure its prey. Its muscles are both strong and compact. Its jaw muscles are especially remarkable for their solidity. Its foot is not in the closed form of a hoof, it is divided and armed with hooked claws. Its teeth are sharp. Indeed everything is adapted to the necessity of surprising and dismembering its prey. The bladder will be smaller in view of the bitterness of its urine that obliges it to be contracted more often in order to empty it. The abdomen will be less salient in view of the small volume of gastric viscera.[9]

The name of Bichat is prominent. Achille-Cléophas quotes Bichat's list of tissue types and offers his own minor corrections. In the spirit of Bichat he proposes 'a convincing proof that some animals need less air than others comes if we put beneath the dome of a pneumatic machine a bird, a small mammal and a reptile. If we then pump out the air the animals will die at different times according to the order indicated.'[10] Evidently, Achille-Cléophas has witnessed, or at least read about, the experiments in physiology conducted in Paris by Bichat. He obviously hasn't seen Bichat in person, but he may well have seen first-generation disciples of Bichat repeating his experiments.

When certain topics come up there is a distinct fugitive imaginative energy in the writing. Here for instance is the description of contractility:

> Contraction of tissues is that faculty which organs have of shrivelling up, of tightening up, of pulling back into themselves, in order to occupy a smaller volume, and they do this gradually, little by little, independently of the will and of any external agency.[11]

In this next passage, Buffon's vision of an amorous world of nature coexists with the more matter-of-fact sensibility of the surgeon:

> The more energetic respiration becomes the more influence it will have; that is why the birds are so prompt and so quick in their loves and why they have such a large number of little ones.[12]

The violence of the revolutionary decade leaves its imprint upon this passage:

> When once a being is deprived of life all the objects that surround it and to which until now it has not succumbed pounce upon it from all sides to exert their power upon it.[13]

And there is a memorable encounter, brief and strange, between the surgeon and the poet in this passage discussing the theme of voluntary movement. It goes far beyond the immediate requirements of the lecture.

> Let your imagination create a being with the power of locomotion and take feeling away from him, he falls over constantly, bumping into everything

around him, he runs continually to his ruin. Imagine on the other hand a second being with feeling. Attached to the soil on which he was born, with no power to escape from that which tends to his destruction, no power to seek out that which serves his pleasure or the sustaining of his life, we shudder at the evils to which he will be exposed. What a deplorable situation, what an unhappy existence! What thing could be more fitting over which to shed our tears? It is a thing to soften the hardest heart, that fiction of an epic poet, that unfortunate Clorinda, shedding her tears along with her blood whilst imprisoned in the bark of a cypress tree. What could be worse for a brave man then to see himself assaulted and not be able to defend himself? It is a horrible thing, a thing of desperation.[14]

The 'fiction of the epic poet', as evoked here, refers to an episode from Book 13 of the sixteenth-century Italian epic *Jerusalem Delivered* by Torquato Tasso. The 'unfortunate Clorinda' is the deceased lover of the quest knight, Tancred. With his sword, Tancred begins to cut down an enchanted cypress tree when the voice of Clorinda reproaches him from within the wounded tree.

In Achille-Cléophas's hands, this episode becomes a parable of the powerfully transgressive dimension of surgical practice. What comes through, carefully displaced into the remote and fanciful discourse of an Italian Renaissance poetic romance, is the story of a haunting. Learning anatomy, we cut into the flesh of the dead and we call it post-mortem dissection. That is safely unambiguous. But then in the next phase, as surgeons, we cut into the flesh and bone of the wide-awake living. We see their pain, but we have learnt to refuse it, to ignore it by 'pretending' that they are dead. The Clorinda episode tells of a terrifying awakening of the imagination to the horror of this confusion between the living and the dead, this benevolent fiction installed in the mind of the surgeon, enabling his hand to work proficiently.

The memory of the poem allows Achille-Cléophas to conduct a brief thought experiment in the tradition of the Enlightenment. If this corpse could speak, what might it say to me? What if this corpse were not some anonymous insentient thing but the body of the woman I love?

Let us follow the Clorinda story in some detail, in the words of Fairfax's translation of Tasso. The knight, Tancred, reaches the cypress grove and is about to cut into the tree when a mysterious inscription warns him not to proceed:

'Oh hardy knight, who through these woods hast passed:
Where Death his palace and his court doth hold!
Oh trouble not these souls in quiet placed,
Oh be not cruel as thy heart is bold' […]

Then he hears a warning voice, which moves him and delays him:

a sound like speech of human kind,
But full of sorrow grief and woe was it,
Whereby his gentle thoughts all filled were
With pity, sadness, grief, compassion, fear.

Tancred ignores the second warning and begins to cut:

He drew his sword at last, and gave the tree
A mighty blow, that made a gaping wound,
Out of the rift red streams he trickling see […]

The voice comes to him once again. This is the third unambiguous warning:

Within this woful cypress laid,
My tender rind thy weapon sharp doth rive,
Cruel, is't not enough thy foes to kill,
But in their graves wilt thou torment them still?

He drops his sword in horror at what he is doing:

Cold and trembling waxed his frozen heart,
Such strange effects, such passions it torment,
Out of his feeble hand his weapon start,
Himself out of his wits nigh, after went: […]

Finally, he sees what he is doing and knows to whom he is doing it. This is not a tree. This is the thing he loves best. In a moment, all his carefully crafted control of emotion is defeated:

Wounded he saw, he thought, for pain and smart,
His lady weep, complain, mourn, and lament,

Nor could he suffer her dear blood to see,
Or hear her sighs that deep far fetched be.

If Achille-Cléophas could see and think and imagine, his 'fierce heart which death had scorned oft' would be moved, and then he, like Tancred, would drop his knife. If this does not happen, except under poetic licence, this is because, as Achille-Cléophas asserts later in his lectures:

The senses, sight, hearing […] the intellectual faculties, none of these can be continuously in action. Habitual sensation blunts feeling. Reflection, imagination cannot be always in motion.[15]

He can identify with Tasso's Tancred in his moment of weakness. However, Achille-Cléophas knows himself to be one of the elect. That knowledge comes through, in the lectures, when he observes, in relation to the training of the senses:

Seeing a picture for the first time a painter will observe numerous details that will escape the attention of other men. In a concert a musician will hear a false note that the rest of the audience are unlikely to notice. How he will excel above those who have never studied, he who from childhood has exercised his intellectual functions, his memory, his judgement.[16]

That final sentence, slipping unawares into autobiography, asserts an implicit moral affinity between the physician, the painter and the musician. They hear and they see things because they have trained their senses. The surgeon combines many exemplary qualities: 'a certain delicacy of all his senses, as well as strength of mind'.[17] For Achille-Cléophas, as early as 1808, the practice of scientific medicine encompasses a distinctive aesthetic and moral experience as well as specialised technical knowledge. To be an enlightened physician is to be a man of compassionate imagination. Remembering his father in later years, Gustave Flaubert praised exactly this quality: 'How often did I hear my father say that he diagnosed people's ailments without knowing how or why'.[18]

ON 27 DECEMBER 1810, just after the end of his fourth year in Rouen, Achille-Cléophas presented his final dissertation to the five examiners of the Paris Faculty of Medicine. The title page is worth quoting here. It describes how medical knowledge was framed.

DISSERTATION NO 103
On the management of the sick before and after surgical operations;
Presented and defended before the Faculty of Medicine in Paris
on 27 December 1810
BY ACHILLE CLEOPHAS FLAUBERT,
born in the town of Meziere in the Department of the Aube,
DOCTOR OF MEDICINE;
Former Pupil of the Ecole practique; former Surgical Intern at the Hotel Dieu in Paris; Assistant Demonstrator in Anatomy at the Hospice d'Humanite in Rouen, in the Department of the Lower Seine.
PRINTED IN PARIS AT THE PRESS OF DIDOT JEUNE
Printer to the Faculty of Medicine, rue des Macons-Sorbonne, n. 13
1810.
TO MY FATHER.
TO MY MASTERS
LAUMONIER AND DUPUYTREN.
This testimony of my warm and sincere gratitude.

Browsing through the seventy printed pages of this modest but elegant volume, we open a small door into the distant medical world of the early nineteenth-century hospital. Four years in Paris, followed by four years in Rouen, have furnished him with an abundance of clinical material. He can now synthesise all that he has learnt from Hallé and from his more recent mentor in Rouen, Laumonier. It has been claimed, by a local historian, a man with a small sharp local axe to grind, that it was in fact Laumonier who devised most of the pre- and post-operative procedures that Achille-Cléophas describes in his thesis.[19] It remains impossible, at this distance, to verify such a claim.

In his dissertation (surprisingly, his only major publication), Achille-Cléophas 'formulated the principles, from which he never departed',[20] a phrase that may suggest either a magisterial consistency or a one-eyed fixity of opinion. He explores what might now be called the psycho-somatic aspects of medicine, all the curious traffic that runs between the body and the mind. His professional ideal is a humane healing wisdom grounded in the best scientific knowledge of his day; his dissertation is accordingly rather different in its scope and its method from other medical dissertations of the same year. The other contemporary dissertations that I have examined were all technical treatises on some specialised aspect of surgery, complete with illustrations and detailed case histories.

Distinctively, Achille-Cléophas combines a precise physiological notation of bodily symptoms with a vividly sympathetic perception of the patient as a fellow-creature, subject to feelings of terror and desire, hope and despair. The physician must not ignore these feelings because they are a significant part of the clinical picture. Drawing upon his own aspirations and upon the example of his masters, Achille-Cléophas portrays a physician who brings many attributes to the task of healing. He must have a knowledge of anatomy, exceptional manual dexterity, a certain *finesse* or delicacy of the five senses, and a real strength of mind. He will observe the temperament and the physical condition of his patient. He will also attend to all the other factors that influence recovery.

Allow the patient, says Achille-Cléophas, to relax for several days beforehand, in the place where the operation is to take place.[21] Keep a special eye on 'debauched' patients. They must be prevented from masturbating. The oversensitive types, who can be recognised by their plumpness and the whiteness of their skin, will benefit from cold baths.[22] Talk to the patient attentively before the operation. Reassure him. Tell him that it will be quick and not very painful. Imaginative patients, especially those who have read medical books, pose a special problem. Their excess of sensibility may become a problem. Anxiety and terror will render them more susceptible to infection. In a state of anxiety the heart beats more slowly, the breathing becomes laboured, the skin goes cold, the muscles relax, sweat covers the body and there is copious diarrhoea. In a state of terror the pulse races, the patient blacks out or bursts into sardonic laughter. Some lose blood. Some have convulsions. All surgical instruments should be concealed from the patient's eyes and you must never discourage the patient from screaming during the operation. The scream always alleviates pain. In the first phase after the operation, the spasm, the patient's skin is dry and cold, the pulse is weak and rapid, all secretions cease, there is shivering and vomiting and the mind itself seems exhausted.[23] In the second phase the skin is warm and damp, the face is pink, breathing is easy, the pulse is strong and regular, the mind revives, blood seeps back into the veins and floods the open wound.[24] After the operation we may give the patient half a glass of wine,[25] remembering to change the patient's blood-stained sweat-soaked shirt as often as necessary. Narcotics such as opium, camphor or quinine can now be used to induce and control sleep.[26] Sunlight will 'augment the vital forces'.[27] Humid air, heavy with 'animal emanations', will increase postoperative mortality.[28]

Finally, the physician is advised to assume a calm and confident manner whenever approaching the patient.[29] In the days before anaesthesia and antisepsis, when surgeons prided themselves on being able to amputate a leg in less than ten seconds, often to polite applause, all these details listed by Achille-Cléophas might well make the difference between life and death.

Achille-Cléophas proclaimed the virtues of scientific medicine. Why should he not? Paris had given him the best medical education in Europe. The medical sensibility that speaks from the pages of his 1810 thesis is sternly materialist, lucidly impersonal and authoritative. But it is obvious, from the testimony of those who had seen Achille-Cléophas at work, that intuition and empathy played a large part in his therapeutic success. Beneath the brilliant rational surface, his mind is responding to deep currents of pity and horror. The same tension between explicit impersonality and unspoken compassion animates the mature style of his son.

ACHILLE-CLÉOPHAS RETURNED TO ROUEN after the success of his thesis in 1810. The diploma that he was carrying entitled him to practice as a doctor of medicine. That diploma was granted 'In the Name of Napoleon, Emperor of the French, King of Italy, and Protector of the Confederation of the Rhine'.[30] In less than five years time, the name of Napoleon would be banished from orthodox public discourse. The diploma would remain, fossil evidence of an era that was increasingly difficult to recall.

By returning to Rouen, Achille-Cléophas was effectively excluding himself from the Parisian medical elite. What lay behind his decision to return? Had his superior, Laumonier, nearing retirement, tempted him with promises of advancement? Or was Achille-Cléophas detained by the prospect of a liaison with Laumonier's young niece, Caroline Fleuriot, the orphaned heiress? Perhaps both inducements were at work.

11

Heiress and Orphan

Like those substances once thought indivisible in which modern scientists, the more closely they examine them, find more and more separate particles, the French bourgeoisie, while seemingly a uniform mass, was extremely composite.
— ALEXIS DE TOCQUEVILLE, *The Old Regime and the French Revolution*
(1856)

MARRY THE MASTER'S DAUGHTER: in a world not yet perfectly rational it remains the classic strategy of self-advancement. Of course, such motives would never have been suggested within the loyal family circle that eventually formed around Achille-Cléophas. The marriage that took place in Rouen in February 1812 between Achille-Cléophas and Caroline Fleuriot was, so they said, all for love. To understand the workings of that marriage, we shall have to read between the lines, attending to the truth of both the social and the sentimental dimensions of a relationship that lasted thirty-four years until the death of the husband. The official fact is that in February 1812, at the age of twenty-seven, Achille-Cléophas married Laumonier's eighteen-year-old ward, the orphaned heiress Caroline Fleuriot. By the time of their marriage, the couple had known each other for about five years, from the time when Caroline had originally arrived in Rouen at the age of thirteen.

The other official fact is that Achille-Cléophas had already resigned from his post as Laumonier's assistant in April 1811, three months after the success of his thesis. For the next four years his name disappears from the hospital archives, and we may assume that he took this opportunity to set up his own medical practice in Rouen. The prospect of his future wife's private income had given him a pleasant freedom of manoeuvre.[1]

Flaubert family tradition made great play of the fact that Caroline Fleuriot was descended, on her mother's side, from the minor aristocracy of Lower Normandy. For Caroline herself, this was a comforting thought, in an early life marked by great adversity. In her romantic version of things, her mother had imprudently married an obscure country doctor. It was 'a most unequal marriage', according to her relatives, who had tried to prevent their union by sequestering the dissident young woman in a convent. She had escaped from the convent, following some piece of nocturnal intrigue worthy of the pages of *Les Liaisons dangereuses.*

The reality of Caroline's early family history was darker and altogether more prosaic. Caroline's paternal great-grandfather had been a linen merchant and a man of property. Her father, Jean-Baptiste Fleuriot, a modest country doctor, having inherited some portion of that fortune, had married above himself. Her mother, Anne Charlotte Cambremer, was the daughter of a rich lawyer, a man with a coat of arms and a seventeenth-century mansion, loathed for his self-importance both by his servants and by those who farmed his land. The wedding between the heiress and the doctor took place in November 1792. The defiantly splendid church ceremony was intended to signify the bride's family's attachment to the good old way of doing things.

Caroline Fleuriot was born in 1793. Her mother died eight days later, leaving the infant in the hands of her grieving father. The unfortunate Jean-Baptiste and his daughter now went to live in the Cambremer mansion with his father-in-law, the lawyer. This was not a happy situation. The local patriots of the day were not sympathetic to rich octogenarian lawyers and the general mood inside the decaying noble mansion was contagiously miserable. To quote Flaubert's biographer Frederick Brown, it 'hardly fostered girlish exuberance […] growing up motherless in large, drafty, wood-panelled rooms that two centuries of damp Norman weather had turned green with mould and stripped of gilt'.[2]

By the law of contraries, the adult Caroline's account of this portion of her childhood was carefully affirmative. As she told it, the grieving young father took the motherless child to his heart and cared for her with a tender affection. Sixty years later, now a grandmother, the aged Caroline 'remembered fondly her father's kisses […] "He undressed me himself every evening […] and put me in my little bed, wanting to replace my mother in every way"'.[3]

Sadly, the devoted father survived only until his daughter was nine years old. Just before he died in 1802, he entrusted his daughter to two women of his acquaintance who promised that they would take care of the girl until she reached the age of marriage. As in any sentimental novel with an implausibly complex plot, the orphan was handed over to the two obliging women. Down on their luck, victims of the Revolution, they had previously taught at Saint-Cyr, the recently abolished royal school for girls. They were now reduced to running a boarding house on the coast at Honfleur. Both women inconsiderately died, some years after assuming the guardianship of Caroline Fleuriot, and the girl was then passed on once again.

Her tutor then sent her to live in Rouen under the care of his sister, Madame Laumonier. Caroline arrived there in 1807 at the age of thirteen and 'within a few months' she had met the man who was to become her husband. It was an honourable mutual love, with promises of marriage. Yet there were several difficulties. She was not yet of marriageable age; he was not yet fully established in his profession. Furthermore, he did not approve of the careless moral tone that prevailed in the Laumonier circle. Elegant, witty and cynical in the high style of the day, the Laumoniers were responsible for Caroline's welfare. She was an heiress. She was on the threshold of puberty. In their frivolous elite fashion, the Laumoniers might collude in her seduction. Thus it was agreed, at Achille-Cléophas's insistence, and perhaps at his expense, that the thirteen-year-old Caroline would remain secluded in the local convent until her marriage, removing her from obvious moral danger. It was the proper thing to do. One protects the value of one's investment.

How was all this experienced, from her side? We can entertain a plausible generic biographical speculation. This was a young girl who had repeatedly lost those who loved her. Her mother, her father and then the two friends of the family, they had all died before their time, abandoning her, passing her on like an awkward parcel and exposing her to the more or less charitable impulses of a world beset by chronic insidious scarcity. Now, in the person of Achille-Cléophas, here was someone who genuinely wanted to keep hold of her.

For the young girl, it signified a thrillingly imperious possessiveness in her suitor. No doubt he impressed her greatly, with his energy, his ambition, his intelligence and his simple, relentless belief in himself. For her part she would be decorously grateful and compliant. A little emotional warmth would be enough to bring her back to life. His admiration would rouse her, little by little, from her frozen state of mourning.

There was also, of course, a significant financial dimension to this marriage. A family council was convened on the eve of the wedding, to establish the legal terms of the marriage contract. According to this contract, the husband could manage but could not inherit his wife's estate. Along with a legitimate pride in her superior social origins, the heiress brought with her a trousseau worth 6,000 francs, some bedroom furniture and some property. She owned a farm situated between Pont l'Évêque and Trouville, yielding an annual income of 4,000 livres. This was a little less than 4,000 francs in 1812, worth around 12,000 pounds sterling in 2012 prices. Scarcely a fortune, it was a useful supplement to the family income. A farm worker might earn around 500 francs a year. The farm brought in eight times that much.

More significantly, this rental income would be sufficient to enfranchise Achille-Cléophas in 1815. Article 40 of the Charter of that year restricted the vote to men of thirty years of age or more who paid at least 300 francs a year in the direct taxes that were levied primarily on revenue from real estate. To meet the tax qualification you needed an annual income of 3,000 to 4,000 francs. Only 80,000 men, 0.3 per cent of the population, met that requirement. On the day of his marriage, whatever else it meant to him, Achille-Cléophas found himself numbered among France's richest men. Passion and calculation were nicely harmonised in a single object of desire. When Achille-Cléophas began to buy land, in the 1830s, his initial purchases would be adjacent to his wife's original farm, the nucleus of the new patrimony.

Along with the income from the farm and the right to vote, marriage to Caroline Fleuriot also brought with it benefits of the less tangible kind. Achille-Cléophas was marrying into the local elite. His new wife was effectively the boss's daughter. If he were prudent and competent, Achille-Cléophas would one day surely inherit the position currently occupied by Laumonier of director of the Hôtel-Dieu.

In the event, he did not have to wait very long. For the moment though, Achille-Cléophas's decision to remain in Rouen appeared to be against his professional interests. He would have done better to return to Paris where the medical elite competed for the very biggest prizes. Why was he absenting himself from that arena? In Flaubert family tradition, as recorded by Caroline's niece, the decision to remain in Rouen was carefully explained as a psychological oddity, the supremely impulsive moment in an existence otherwise governed by rational calculation.

Here is that narrative. Based on first-hand conversations with her grandmother, it probably reflects the elderly widow's fond memory of what her husband had told her about the romance of their union.

> Instead of staying a couple of months, the young doctor stayed there all his life. The frequent appeals of numerous friends, the hope of attaining a high position in Paris, a hope justified by his early achievements, nothing persuaded him to leave his hospital and the people to whom he had become deeply attached. But love was the initial reason for this extended stay, love for a girl he glimpsed one morning, a child of thirteen, Madame Laumonier's goddaughter, an orphan who lived in lodgings and came to visit her godmother every week. [...] She had just arrived [...] when they first met; a few months later they confessed their love and exchanged promises.[4]

If this was indeed how he always told it to her, then it was a loyal and affectionate compliment. The truth was evidently more complicated.

THE FIRST HOME, the first love, the first child, those fleeting early years were for husband and wife also an initiation into the proper social pleasures of their time and place. They were becoming cheerfully *bourgeois*, at a time when the word was not yet burdened with its many later negations. Social relations with an almost precisely equivalent bourgeois family were soon established. Caroline's closest friend from her convent days, Marie Victoire Thurin, the beautiful, stylish daughter of a rich ship-owner from Le Havre, had been married in the same year and was living a few miles away in Darnetal.

Marie Victoire had married a local 'industrialist'. The word was still so new that one pronounced it with an air of careless sophistication. His name was Paul Le Poittevin. He was in textiles and he had done well. He was a man who, rather like Achille-Cléophas, had come up from nothing. Born the son of a miller in Bricquebec, a tiny village near the coast, Paul Le Poittevin arrived in Rouen around the year 1800. By 1807 he was foreman in a dye works. He went into business on his own account, married prudently, expanded into weaving and prospered hugely.[5]

The two families formed the perfect alliance. The wives were already friends. For Caroline that friendship was a preciously positive thing, salvaged from a childhood spoilt by sorrow. In due course the liberal industrialist and the medical man became godfathers to each other's children. They had so much in common: modest provincial origin, modernising energy and indifference towards religion. Apart from the private pleasures of mutual family visiting, there were the gratifying public rituals of sociability to be enjoyed.

In the 1820s, Cours-la-Reine, the long tree-lined avenue that ran along the left bank of the river, was the favourite place for *le Tout-Rouen* to go on Sundays. For the evenings there was the Théâtre des arts, a palatial late eighteenth-century building, on a prime site down near the river. One of the best provincial theatres in the country, it had an auditorium large enough for almost two thousand. Specialising in the noble genres for an affluent and educated audience, the theatre maintained separate resident companies, one for drama and one for opera. There were five performances a week, all through a season that ran from the beginning of September until the end of April. It was good form to do the whole repertoire and see popular pieces several times over.[6]

The inner world of any moderately happy marriage is rarely for the telling. Only one or two distinct scenes from this enduring marriage have been preserved, and they point to curiously opposed themes. In this first scene we can observe the earliest years of their marriage. The couple set up house in the heart of the old city, in the busy merchant quarter, on the rue du Petit-Salut, a short narrow street of tall houses, just a few yards away from the cathedral square. Their first child, Achille, is born here. He arrives in the world most auspiciously, on the eve of the first anniversary of their marriage.

For Caroline Flaubert, this is the best time, these years in the first house on the rue du Petit-Salut. In her long widowed old age she would often pass by and look back upon the happiness she had known there. 'In my childhood,' said her granddaughter, 'she often took me that way and she would look at the windows and she would say to me in a solemn almost religious voice, "Look, up there, that's where I spent the best years of my life."'

After the happy birth of their first child in 1813, the couple's reproductive history took a much darker turn. Their next three children all died in early childhood. Caroline died at twenty months; Emile died at eight months; Jules died aged three. To add to Caroline's distress, early in 1818, on the death of Laumonier, the couple moved from their first home on the rue du Petit-Salut to the residential wing of the Hôtel-Dieu where Achille-Cléophas was installed as director of surgery.

Achille-Cléophas probably welcomed the move. Living over the shop meant that he could monitor his patients at all hours of the day and night. Caroline probably deplored it for the very same reason. It removed the boundary between home and work. It placed her and her young family unpleasantly near to traumatic scenes of pain and death. The sounds and the smells of suffering humanity were inescapable. Between the family dining room and the surgical ward there was only a thin wooden partition.

We catch a later glimpse of this marriage in the course of a letter that Gustave Flaubert wrote to his mistress Louise Colet in September 1846, eight months after his father's death. It describes a curious incident from Gustave's childhood:

> I do remember about ten years ago, when we were on holiday, we were all in Le Havre. My father discovered that a woman he had known in his younger days, when he was seventeen, was living there with her son who was now an actor in the theatre there. […] He decided he would go and see her. This woman, a famous beauty in her hometown, had been his mistress in the old days. He did not do what most bourgeois men would do; he did not hide it away. He was too superior for that. So he went to pay her a visit. My mother and the three of us stood outside in the street waiting for him, and the visit lasted nearly an hour.[7]

Beyond the obvious fact that Gustave is idealising his father's somewhat egocentric conduct, the story illuminates, briefly but vividly, the later workings of the marriage. His wife can be expected to wait for him in the street, with the children, for nearly an hour as he catches up, conversationally, with his former mistress. If such things were indeed 'perfectly normal' then this suggests a perfectly compliant wife, loyal to her lord, accepting her subordination without protest.

Such good behaviour came at a certain price. In the early 1840s, during the final few years of her married life, Caroline was much troubled by migraines. Family letters from that period often close with remarks on the intensity and the frequency of her headaches. Characteristically, she is in a bad temper with the cook. She takes to her bed at four in the afternoon. She is half asleep in her chair, her forehead smeared with laudanum.[8]

The final word on Caroline's moral character should come from her son, Gustave. In the year 1852 he described his widowed mother, briefly and enigmatically, to his by then ex-mistress Louise Colet:

> She is very difficult to please. Her whole person expresses something imperturbable, glacial and naïve that is quite disconcerting. She gets by without principles even more readily than without effusions. Though essentially virtuous, she shamelessly declares that she does not know what virtue is and has never had to sacrifice anything to it.[9]

No images of Caroline Fleuriot, either as a child or as a young woman, have survived. The earliest image of her dates from the year 1831 when she was in her late thirties and had given birth to six children in twelve years. A portrait sketch in pencil, it is not very flattering. It depicts a woman swathed up to the chin. She has a small unsmiling mouth and a small head on a large shapeless body.[10]

12

Loyalties

A feeling of extreme uneasiness began to ferment in all young hearts. Condemned to inaction by the powers that governed the world, delivered to vulgar pedants of every kind, to idleness and to ennui, the youth saw the foaming billows that they had prepared to meet subside. All these gladiators, glistening with oil, felt in the bottom of their souls an insupportable wretchedness. The richest became libertines; those of moderate fortune followed some profession.

— ALFRED DE MUSSET, *The Confession of a Child of the Century* (1836)

PARIS, MARCH 1794. The marquis de Condorcet had been in hiding for nearly six months in the safe house on the rue Servandoni. Spring was coming and it was time for him to leave. His protector, Madame Vernet, was in real danger. Already enfeebled by his long seclusion, he had to escape before it was too late. In every city the Revolution was devouring its own, and the name of Condorcet was on the latest list of traitors. Too well-known and too well-liked for public execution, Condorcet suspected that they would poison him, on the quiet, if they ever caught him. Murder your critics; that was the essential logic of the Terror.[1]

Condorcet had spent the long winter months writing his great testimony to the emancipatory powers of reason, *Sketch for a Historical Picture of the Progress of the Human Mind*. In that text, only published after his death, Condorcet asserts that there are 'the strongest grounds for believing that nature has set no limit to our hopes'. He describes a future world 'in which stupidity and misery will at last be only accidental rather than the habitual condition of part of society.'[2] Undaunted, his imagination reaches boldly into the future:

> The time will come when the sun shines only on free human beings who recognise no other master but their reason; when tyrants and slaves, priests and their benighted or hypocritical minions exist only in the history books and the theatre, and our only concern with them is to pity their victims and their dupes, maintain a useful vigilance motivated by horror at their excesses, and know how to recognise and stifle, by the weight of reason, the first seeds of superstition and tyranny that ever dare to reappear.[3]

There was a certain grimly irrefutable irony in Condorcet's situation. The mind was free to imagine a perfect future for the human race. The body was threatened with imminent destruction. The theory and the practice of Enlightenment could scarcely be more askew.

ROUEN, MARCH 1802. Winter drags on and price of bread is up. Forty-three centimes for a big loaf, the *pain bourgeois*. Hungry crowds mean trouble and hordes of beggars have invaded the cathedral. They are unpleasant to the nose. They are troubling to the conscience. They are 'provoking disorder'. Fortified by this happy phrase, the newly appointed archbishop, Étienne Hubert de Cambaceres, well-known for the sumptuousness of his table, announces a robust new church policy on begging. Henceforth, only those wearing the large numbered metal badges given out by the church authorities will be allowed to beg inside the cathedral.

Condorcet in hiding, Cambaceres in power: these two scenes, encapsulate something of the essential moral history of the generation that came of age around the year 1800. They had tasted the wine of revolution. They had listened to intoxicatingly eloquent speeches on the themes of reason and justice and perfectibility. They had seen all the deadly mutual enmity of those impatient to realise that vision. Latterly, they have attended sermons expounding the religious duty of compassion and charity. Leaving church, they have seen the undeserving poor driven from the door. The more imaginative have wondered at the damage that goes with this century of marvels. Over a good meal they have told each other that one day, in the future, things would be better. Some great collective initiative would transform the material and moral conditions of life. There would be education, justice and progress. In the present, though, what is one to do? In the first decades of this new century, in the raw factory towns of the new industrial order, the lucky few are getting rich, but the unlucky seem to be dying ever younger.

As the old sense of a better future faded away, so the present unease went underground. Novels and newspapers nourished an unhappy middle-class fascination with violent crime. According to the influential thesis of the historian Louis Chevalier, the urban working class was henceforth perceived, from above, as the Dangerous Class.[4] The lethally dysfunctional qualities of the modern industrial city incited anxious collective imaginings, both political and literary. There was a new urban imagery of hidden tunnels used by secret societies, a whole world hidden down in the sewers, labyrinthine enclaves of filth and disease where criminal conspiracies were hatched by a feral underclass. Though the Chevalier position has been challenged,[5] the evidence for Rouen suggests that his thesis is largely correct.[6]

THE EVER-IMPENDING SOCIAL QUESTION was not immediately on the agenda when, every Wednesday afternoon, whatever the current political regime, the five eminent men of the Administrative Commission came together around the big table to oversee the complex affairs of the Hôtel-Dieu. Lawyers, merchants and manufacturers, these were men of the class deferentially referred to as *les notables*. They were irreproachably loyal to the government of the day. Proposed for this charitable office by the mayor, approved by the prefect and nominated by the minister in Paris, each man served for five years. During that time, they managed the budget, scrutinised medical education and appointed the senior medical staff, including the chief surgeon.[7]

In the spring of 1815, the Commission was currently attempting to solve a problem of succession at the very top of the Hôtel-Dieu. The health of the chief surgeon, Laumonier, was visibly failing. He should be replaced as soon as possible. However, a little local difficulty had arisen. The local prefect, intent on advertising his zeal to the new regime in Paris, was pushing a mediocre royalist candidate. Laumonier, equally wary of offending the newly installed monarchy, had endorsed the royalist mediocrity as his successor. The Commission thus found itself at an impasse, confronted by an unsuitable candidate being promoted for political reasons.

On 8 March 1815, the Commission unanimously offered the post
of deputy surgeon to Achille-Cléophas.[8] At that point, they must have
known that Napoleon had just escaped from his exile on the island of
Elba and was said to be heading rapidly northwards, across France, in
the direction of Paris. The Commission did not yet know what might be
the outcome, but the timing of their offer to Achille-Cléophas suggests
that they were gambling on the possibility that Napoleon would unseat
Louis XVIII, thus allowing them to snub the royalist mediocrity, without
attracting retribution from above. Seven days earlier, on 1 March 1815,
Napoleon had landed on the French Mediterranean coast, near Antibes.
He was in the city of Lyon by 13 March, and he entered Paris on 20 March,
by which time Louis XVIII had fled.

The Napoleonic interregnum, known as the Hundred Days, was about
to coincide with a perfectly obscure but nicely parallel Flaubertian interregnum, as Achille-Cléophas struggled to have his appointment confirmed. The Commission at the Hôtel-Dieu were told that their initial
procedure was improper. There would have to be a shortlist of three
candidates. Given the extraordinary uncertainties of those months, the
manoeuvring for position, the sudden tactical switching of loyalties, the
mysterious indisposition of senior officers of state, it was not clear how
the problem of the surgical appointment could be resolved. Between May
and November of that year, the city of Rouen got through three mayors,
one of whom lasted for only eleven days. Everyone was playing for time,
even though, with hundreds of wounded soldiers arriving at the Hôtel-
Dieu, the new appointment was urgent.

The situation was further complicated by the fact that Achille-Cléophas
and Laumonier had apparently become estranged at some point. Achille-
Cléophas had resigned from his original position at the Hôtel-Dieu in
April 1811, only a few months after becoming fully qualified. The School
of Artificial Anatomy, set up in 1806, was about to be closed down, for
want of students and lack of cash. Though Achille-Cléophas's resignation
from the Hôtel-Dieu may have been prompted either by Laumonier's
refusal to step aside for him or to promote him or by his reluctance to
let him marry Caroline.

The Commission duly met, as required, with a new shortlist. Once
again they chose Achille-Cléophas as deputy. Ministerial approval
of their choice came through by the end of May. By the end of June
wounded soldiers from the Battle of Waterloo were arriving in their

hundreds at the Hôtel-Dieu. As well as French casualties, there were Prussians, Russians and English among the wounded. Such was the emergency that bandages had to be improvised from the shirts of dead soldiers.

A letter dated 28 June 1815, from Achille-Cléophas to a friend in Paris, informs us that he and Laumonier have settled their differences. 'Before setting foot in the Hôtel-Dieu I have made my peace with Monsieur Laumonier, who assures me that he is content that I have been chosen for the post. We see each other every day, I am full of respect for him [...] he has proposed that I take on the major surgical operations – and it is said by the staff that he is much more cheerful since I have been in the hospital.'[9] In the background of this happier scene, there was great uncertainty. Laumonier's precarious state of health and Napoleon's possible political fate would both influence what happened next, professionally, to Achille-Cléophas.

By the end of the summer Laumonier had fallen into a coma 'after several attacks of apoplexy which have deprived him of his intellectual faculties.'[10] Once again, for the second time in less than a year, the Commission went through the motions of shortlisting candidates. Finally, on 29 November, Achille-Cléophas Flaubert was appointed as chief surgeon. Everyone accepted Achille-Cléophas's judicious proposal that Laumonier be allowed to retain the title, the salary and the lodgings for the remainder of his life. One week later, at the next meeting of the Commission, Achille-Cléophas was ceremoniously installed in the job that he had, in fact, already been doing since March.

He had prevailed by playing his hand carefully. He kept quiet during the Hundred Days, mastering any temptation to share his reasonable delight at the return of Napoleon. When the wheel turned again, after Waterloo, and after the inevitable local purging of those who had sided with the 'usurper', Achille-Cléophas emerged from the shadows, undamaged, and professionally secure. In August 1815, with the Bourbons restored for the second time, Achille-Cléophas submitted his plans for managing the surgical service at the Hôtel-Dieu. He also found time to write a fastidiously apolitical inaugural speech on being invited to join the local Academy. In the near future, there would be other royalists cluttering the immediate landscape, and some of them would undoubtedly be mediocre.

MEANWHILE THERE WAS THE OFFICIAL CEREMONY of appointment,
recorded in some detail, in the archives of the Hôtel-Dieu. Listening in
to those proceedings, we can pick up both the individual voices and the
collective values that they affirm. The president of the Commission on
that day, standing in for the mayor, was the marquis de Martainville. The
son of an aristocratic cavalry officer from one of Normandy's ruling families, the marquis was only a year older than Achille-Cléophas. A man of
immense wealth, and civic energy, mayor of Rouen from 1821 until 1830,
Martainville was strongly attached to the House of Bourbon. Among the
mayors of Rouen, Martainville was the aristocratic anomaly. Since 1790,
all the mayors had all been drawn from the bourgeois merchant community. In this decorous formal encounter between merit and privilege,
between Dr Flaubert and the marquis de Martainville, the whole imperative unhappy post-Restoration politics of coexistence can be observed.

The first portion of the proceedings was conducted before a small
invited audience of surgical colleagues: the interns, the students and the
aspirants. The secretary of the Commission read out the official letters
received from the local prefect and from the minister of the interior.
Then Achille-Cléophas took an oath. This was not the traditional oath
of loyalty to the monarchy, but simply a moral declaration: 'to perform
all tasks faithfully and well, with all the humanity, the commitment, the
zeal and the exactitude that such an important position required.'[11] It is
not clear whether they were using the previous secular oath out of inertia,
or whether that secular oath was deliberately retained as a concession to
the candidate's known sensitivities.

After the oath, the marquis de Martainville delivered his speech. It is
a ripe and corpulent specimen of the official discourse of the hour, with
its double negatives, its dilated presidential syntax and its decorous ideal-
isations. But it is also of real interest for what it says, in this first section,
both about the official social mission of the Hôtel-Dieu and about the
acknowledged public character of Achille-Cléophas.

> The administration of the hospices of this town, whose active and paternal
> solicitude touches upon everything of consequence to these great and valu-
> able establishments, where the ailing and the indigent, the abandoned child,
> and the destitute elderly find a refuge and a comfort, the administration has
> felt for some time the need to restore to the surgical service in the *hospice
> d'humanité* [still the official title] all that has been lacking due to the absence

of the chief surgeon, where, in spite of the zealous efforts of the resident students to alleviate the effects of this absence, both clinical medicine and medical teaching could not fail to be adversely affected. It is to bring this state of affairs to an end that the administration has solicited on your behalf, Monsieur, your appointment as deputy to Monsieur Laumonier, and that we have finally obtained from the government your definitive appointment to this important position. It is thanks to the solid knowledge, thanks to the talents of which you have already given evidence, talents which did not escape the vigilant eye of the administration, when you were formerly employed here; it is also thanks to the well-deserved reputation that you have acquired since then, a reputation in advance of your years; it is thanks to all these that you are now the one who is honourably chosen: a choice which you will justify on every occasion. The unfortunate will always find in you the compassion that will enhance the resources of your art in helping them to bear their ills more patiently.'[12]

Martainville then expounds to Achille-Cléophas his duty to ensure decorum in the treatment of the corpses that will provide the material of his anatomy lessons. Here we encounter a local version of those larger cultural anxieties concerning dissection rooms and the proper treatment of dead bodies. It can be argued that from the year 1815 a new regime was in the making. After so many bodies in pieces, after so many memories of violence to be banished from the national memory, there had to be a sterner decorum observed, henceforth, in all those places where bodies, living or dead, could legitimately be taken apart. The historian Robert Tombs has suggested that three contemporary cultural initiatives were connected by this undeclared agenda: 'Medical dissection of corpses was removed from the public gaze. It became ever more difficult to get into the morgue. Public executions were moved to quieter places and daybreak. The guillotine was taken down from its platform and placed less visibly on the ground.'[13]

In this spirit of greater discretion, Martainville lays out both the problem and the expected solution. Essentially, Achille-Cléophas will be trusted to police the behaviour of his medical students.

If, for the public good, there were any need to arouse and sustain a zeal less enlightened and less eager than your own, I would mention as exemplary those eminent men who have preceded you in this same position. I would quote the name of the celebrated Lecat, a name that remains one of the glories of this institution, a man who was such a credit to the art that he professed, who first introduced into Rouen that style of teaching so effective in aiding the progress of science, by means of expert demonstrations of practical anatomy, at which he could extract from the cold carcass of a man deprived of life the secret knowledge that would alleviate the sufferings of the living man and prolong his existence. What difficulties did he have to overcome in order to set up and sustain this useful facility, mostly by reason of the prejudices hostile to the advancement of the art of anatomy; prejudices not in themselves dishonourable, since they arose from a religious respect for the dead. In the anatomy lessons which you, Monsieur, will teach for the education of your students, you will not have to struggle, as he did in those times now long gone, with the same obstacles. Perhaps, in place of that excessive respect for the dead, you may have to repress the contrary excess that has become all too common in amphitheatres and anatomy laboratories where dissections are carried out and where thoughtless youth, who do not yet have any sense of the dignity of man, sometimes engage in scandalous behaviour, in a species of impiety towards the lifeless form of a being who once breathed and was perhaps blessed with qualities lacking in those who so disrespect his remains. The strictness of your moral principles will not allow you to tolerate indecent abuses of any kind: the excellent qualities of your heart, which are so in harmony with your distinctively modest excellence, these things are a sure guarantee of the harmony that will reign continually in the relations that you will have with all persons attached to this hospital: you will show the unfailing respect that is their due to those respectable women whom providence appears to have created specially to help and comfort suffering humanity. Finally, you will fulfil the expectations of the administration by even surpassing its hopes.[14]

Achille-Cléophas makes his brief conventional response to the president's speech. The audience leaves the room, and the Commission goes into private session with Achille-Cléophas. Having rehearsed the high-minded preliminaries, it was now time to spell out to Achille-Cléophas the precise conditions of his employment. These conditions are listed as eighteen numbered paragraphs, like a formal legal contract. Reading between the lines, we can reconstruct something of what had been happening, during the recent emergency, as well as what was supposed to happen in future, in the Hôtel-Dieu.

As chief surgeon, Achille-Cléophas is to be continuously responsible for instructing his students. (This implies that medical education had languished under Laumonier.) He is required to give written notice to the Commission when he proposes to begin a course of anatomy lessons. He is not permitted to take or to request payment from any of his students.

He is not allowed to 'take from its bed immediately after death any human body without having first informed the Mother Superior [...] in order to confirm whether or not this cadaver will be required by the family and whether or not the procedures relative to this death have been carried out.' (In view of the recent emergency conditions of confusion and overcrowding, it seems likely that the corpses had gone astray, and that there had been conflicts between nuns and surgeons over the proper management of human remains.) Achille-Cléophas is not allowed to remove from the mortuary any cadaver to which is attached a card indicating that the body has been claimed by the family; he shall only be allowed to engage in those investigations that enable him to establish and to document the causes of death; however he is required to reassemble and stitch body parts back together, covering the corpse so that the eye is not surprised nor the heart stricken, when the nuns enter to perform the last rites.

We may picture some of the unfortunate scenes that this clause was intended to avoid. The regulation of the entire process had evidently been chaotic, latterly, under Laumonier. Corpses legitimately obtained must also be correctly managed. To this end, interestingly elaborate procedures are proposed.

In order to satisfy the requirements of instruction as well as to remedy the abuses that arise from too ready a supply of cadavers, only one cadaver per week will normally be delivered for dissection, from the first day of October until the last day of April. (In the years before the invention of artificial refrigeration systems, dissections were normally confined to the cold winter months.) If more cadavers are required, this shall only be with the explicit authorisation of the director of the Hôtel-Dieu. The porter shall make no deliveries of cadavers without joint written authorisation from the chief surgeon and the director. The chief surgeon shall be responsible for the shrouds supplied and will ensure that cadavers delivered to him are returned for the purposes of burial. He shall ensure that the cadavers do not remain too long in the laboratory; that body parts are not scattered here and there; that body parts are carefully reassembled once the procedures to which they are subject have been completed, in order to avoid all risk of putrefaction. He shall not allow any intern or any student to remove any anatomical specimen without the consent of the administration.

All major surgical operations, especially those involving fractures, shall be carried out by Achille-Cléophas. Under his direct supervision, he shall be allowed to delegate surgical tasks to an intern of proven capacity. Students shall bleed patients only in the presence of Achille-Cléophas or of an intern. Only the interns shall bleed the women in the labour ward, which ward students are strictly forbidden to enter. The chief surgeon is to inspect all wounds and dressings. He is to ensure the presence in the building, day and night, of the duty intern. He is to ensure that dressings are completed promptly, in order to avoid the abuses arising from students lingering over the task.

Every three months, Achille-Cléophas is to submit to the Commission a detailed report on all the surgical staff under his management, both students and interns. No more than twenty students are to be employed in the surgical division at any one time. Laumonier had admitted more than fifty students. Though this dealt with the recent clinical emergency, it was regarded from above as ruinously expensive. Laumonier, for all his talents, had proved increasingly chaotic in his administration of the service. It was expected that Achille-Cléophas would be more consistently in command of the details.

He met their expectations in full. Order was restored. In the first five years, all of his structural proposals, for interns and for students, were accepted without question by the Commission. He acquired extensive powers of patronage, as well as powers of censure over unruly subordinates. In 1819, for instance, when students protested at his dismissal of three of their number, the Commission came down heavily on them. In accord with his own energetic ethos, Achille-Cléophas encouraged emulation and 'the noble sentiment of ambition' among his interns and his students. There was to be a competition for the coveted internships. There was to be an annual prize ceremony for the students, to reward good progress and good behaviour.[15]

Laumonier died in January 1818. At that point, as agreed, Achille-Cléophas came into his own. Twelve years after arriving in Rouen, he finally stepped into the title, the salary and the lodgings of the chief surgeon.

THE PROLIFICALLY SUCCESSFUL PATTERN of Achille-Cléophas's life will continue all through his thirties. Then on a summer evening in 1825, his fortieth year, good fortune deserts him. He is travelling in his carriage along a country road, returning from a consultation. It is around nine in the evening and there are still several hours of daylight. Thirty kilometres from home, his carriage runs out of control on a dangerous hill. He jumps out to save himself and fractures his left leg as he lands on the ground. His life is in danger: the upper fragment of the tibia has pierced the skin.

In great pain, as the fractured leg began to swell, Achille-Cléophas was carried to the nearby Chateau Mauny. There, in the words of the newspaper report, he was 'the object of the most compassionate attention from the marquis d'Etampes and his family.' During the following day and night, the swelling increased, the fever continued and the skin on the leg became covered in blisters. Rumours of his imminent death began to circulate in Rouen: 'The interest that is generally taken in the person of Monsieur Flaubert means that every account of his current condition is taken up avidly. Information that several alarming symptoms had appeared [...] have increased public anxiety for the life of this friend of humanity.'

Over the next few days, Achille-Cléophas's deputy surgeon, Dr Leudet, took it upon himself to write daily bulletins for the *Journal de Rouen*. He confounded the rumours and praised the courage displayed by the victim of the accident. These are fascinating texts, for the sincerely heroic moral tale that they propagate. In Leudet's account, the physician-turned-patient sustains his exemplary public character. In the face of his own death, the friend of humanity is lucidly resourceful, tenderly considerate of his wife, conscientiously supportive of his colleague. He is a man in a great tradition that reaches back across the centuries. Dr Leudet tells the story:

> It is difficult to have any notion of the calm which M. Flaubert has preserved in the midst of the atrocious pain caused by his fracture. Whilst waiting for the arrival of M. Licquet, doctor of medicine, and one of his former pupils whose presence he had requested, he prepared part of the apparatus designed to hold the fractured limb, after which he wrote a fairly long letter to his wife, informing her of the accident, though with an exemplary restraint intended to make the news less painful, conveying a positive hope that he did not actually feel.

As the fracture was being set, he helped Dr Licquet with his advice, showing all the composure and precision that he would himself have shown if he had been dealing with a patient. Here is yet one more affinity between Monsieur Flaubert and the famous surgeon Ambroise Paré. The latter also had a fractured leg, and likewise gave the doctor who was binding it the most sage advice delivered with the most admirable composure.[16]

As Achille-Cléophas recovered, his accident disappeared from the news, pushed aside by copiously detailed reports of local celebrations for the coronation of King Charles X. Though Achille-Cléophas survived, his general health may have been slowly compromised by the damage to his leg. In 1841 his nine-year-old son Gustave writes to a schoolfriend reassuring him that his father, Achille-Cléophas, has now recovered from an episode of severe rheumatism during which he was unable to walk.[17]

13

Future Perfect

AMONG THE VARIOUS LEARNED SOCIETIES that flourished in the city of Rouen, the most exclusive, the most prestigious and the most conservative was the Académie des sciences, belles lettres et arts de Rouen. Founded in 1744, it was a provincial version of the Académie française. Abolished in 1793 and restored in 1803, by the late summer of 1815, when Achille-Cléophas became a member, the Rouen Academy was *royale* once again.

Supplanting the aristocratic salon, such academies were formally egalitarian enclaves of high-minded, secular masculine culture, both scientific and literary. The men of the academies saw themselves, flatteringly, as the bourgeois children of the Enlightenment. They had dedicated themselves to science, to the collective pursuit of social improvement through science. They were doing serious, modern, useful stuff, as opposed to the trivial pursuits of women and noblemen.[1]

Whatever its modernising mission, the Rouen Academy visibly retained certain links to the past. Among its cherished customs, there was an annual prize essay competition. The essay committee set the topic and there was a handsome silver medal, value three hundred francs, for the winner. The prize medals, for this period, depict Minerva enthroned. She is pointing up towards a classical temple set on a hill. Her Latin motto is TRIA LIMINA PANDIT. *She opens three doors*: the doors being the three divisions of knowledge specified in the Academy's formal title. Achille-Cléophas was a member of the Academy's prize committee in 1824, when the proposed essay topic was 'The Therapeutic Value of Leeches'.[2]

Membership of the Rouen Academy was limited to fifty. You became a member only by invitation, after a ceremonial sequence of votes, visits and speeches. There were weekly meetings on Friday evenings, meetings at which members reported formally on the latest discoveries in their field. Individual reports were included in full in the Academy's annual transactions. This was a handsome, substantial, subsidised volume that affirmed the social status rather than the intellectual ambition of its contributors.

The typical annual volume from the years between 1815 and 1830 is a curious mixture of science, antiquarianism, inaugural speeches and poetry reviews, along with a lengthy and resplendently turgid annual address from the president of the Academy. The inflated style, whatever its comic resonance, is evidence of an exceptionally vigorous moral consensus among the assembled members. The Academy was evidently both a convivial evening with the boys and a glorious Arena of Fraternal Emulation.

The Rouen Academy was an arena in which Achille-Cléophas was going to feel at home. He had always thrived on fraternal emulation. For men of his generation, serious masculine identity was powered by emulation. Emulation was both Republican and Napoleonic. It was invigorating, a positive stimulus to virtue, a pure form of rivalry that had ideally been cleansed of envy. Such was at least the theory of emulation.

Studying a series of those annual Rouen Academy volumes, we can observe the workings of that distant social world. Most of the published reports are scientific, and they are grouped together under a dozen headings, according to discipline. The reports for 1817 include astronomy, mechanics, physics, natural history, zoology, botany, geology, entomology, chemistry, human medicine, veterinary medicine and agriculture. The largest category is medical, being a subject of the most immediate utility. Typically there may be a dozen medical reports in a single year.

The current, resident members of the Academy are listed at the end of each volume. Their occupations, their inaugural year and their public honours are carefully spelt out. For the year 1827, in a list of some thirty members, we find the following occupations listed: two national deputies, one royal councillor, the local prefect, one senior employee from the Prefecture, two physicians (both in senior positions at the Hôtel-Dieu), two lawyers, one senior judge, one high-ranking army officer with the title of count, one marquis, one merchant, one cider-maker, two senior members of the church, the local archbishop, the city architect, the city engineer, the city tax officer, the city archivist, the director of the local mint, the director of the botanical garden, one antiquary, one veterinarian, one horologist, three science teachers and one society painter.[3]

The social composition of this elite body is fascinating. The membership list tells us a great deal about how social status and cultural authority were distributed in Rouen in the late 1820s. Senior members of the liberal professions form the miscellaneous majority. The aristocracy, the church and the army are included, but they are not dominant. There is only one merchant on the list. The modernising liberal–professional majority appears to be at ease with the elder powers of aristocracy, church and army. On the other hand, the big new money, from the factories and the mills, has not yet been consecrated.

That ethos, poised between the old and the new, is succinctly expressed in this passage, taken from the president's annual address of 1817:

> It is a splendid thing, of interest to all classes in society, this meeting of men who, in the sole hope of being useful, with no other end than the public good and the general interest of society, dedicate themselves to the most difficult researches, to the most abstract meditations, the most arduous undertakings, in order to nourish the love of letters, to encourage the taste for science, to accelerate the progress of the arts, to excite emulation and to develop talent of every kind.[4]

ACHILLE-CLÉOPHAS GAVE HIS INAUGURAL ADDRESS to the Academy in August 1815. A richly suggestive text, both succinct and ambitious, it distils the Enlightenment aspiration to perfectibility expressed in the work of Buffon, Condorcet, Bichat, Cuvier and Cabanis. It is a manifesto for 'interdisciplinary' scientific medicine. I shall quote the full text, interpolating my commentary in italics.

> Monsieur Flaubert, Doctor of Medicine, admitted to share in the work of the Academy, delivered his inaugural address.
>
> After having thanked the Academy for having given him a place among its Members, our new colleague endeavoured to establish the numerous close links between medicine and all branches of human knowledge.
>
> Metaphysics, said Monsieur Flaubert, offers the physician that valuable method of analysis without which he is the plaything of pathological disorders, just as the pilot of a ship without sail or compass is subject to the caprice and the fury of the winds. *This is a nice opening flourish. It advertises the speaker's ability to deploy the rich figurative powers of language. It notifies*

*his audience that he shares their regard for the aesthetic. It announces an
educated man with a generous surplus of cultural capital behind him. Achille-
Cléophas is of the generation for whom the language of medical science is still
allowed to be richly figurative.* Metaphysics purifies language by rectifying
ideas; only if he walks by the light of this torch can the physician hope to
treat delirium, mania, hypochondria, melancholy and all such disorders of
the organ of thought.

*That phrase, organ of thought, is highly significant. It denies the soul. It
points to Cabanis.*

The study of moral philosophy, that science which teaches us to control our passions to some proper end, is no less necessary for all who
profess the art of healing. This it is which indicates the means we must
employ against the moral disorders that we encounter. Here is a man fallen
from the very summit of greatness. He must be brought round to simpler
tastes, to more modest desires. Here is an ambitious man. He must be
cured of the fatal passion that is devouring him. Here is a miser. He must
learn to open his heart to the needs of the poor. These parents, be they
selfish, stupid or prejudiced, must be won over in order to save the life
of a young girl who has fallen victim of an innocent love. *The physician is
no mere technician. He is the friend of humanity, the licensed moral agent
of the highest collective values.* This grieving mother, weeping at the grave
of her husband, her only son, her beloved daughter, she must be comforted and consoled, taught by Religion to picture a happy future for her
dear departed who dwells already in the eternal mansion set aside for the
pure in heart.

*Achille-Cléophas is treading carefully here. He knows his present audi-
ence. On their account, he eschews the reflex Voltairean mockery of religious
belief. His grieving mother, comforted by her belief in the afterlife, is pictured
compassionately but with a carefully muted scepticism. As if to say, we as educated men do not share her faith, but we can see that her faith is good for her.
This is a characteristic nineteenth-century psychological pattern: the poetry
of religion is fine for women. We men are made of sterner stuff. And perhaps
Achille-Cléophas is reassuring an all-male audience, by whom he wishes to
be accepted, that he is not a godless materialist.*

Jurisprudence plays its part in the art of healing. It serves to guide the
physician in the exercise of legal medicine. But it is above all in the physical
sciences that the physician can hope to find the most powerful means, both
useful and necessary in the exercise of his art.

Geology will show him the changes that floods, the great catastrophes of the Earth, have wrought in the human constitution.

Meteorology will instruct him in the levels of heat and cold, dryness or humidity and atmospheric pressure that are harmful or beneficial to the development and the exercise of the functions of the human body.

Statics and dynamics will teach him to calculate the power of the muscles.

Optics will reveal to him the secrets of the action of light, whether direct, reflected or refracted, upon the eye; as well as giving him the certain means to remedy the disorders which can affect that admirable organ of vision.

Admirable organ of vision: a classic periphrasis.

Physics is especially useful to the surgeon in the treatment of injuries, their effects, fractures and dislocations; as well as in the construction, the improvement and the use of his instruments.

What a truly immense fund of knowledge does chemistry offer to the physician! The nature and the properties, whether useful or harmful, of the different gases; the composition of the air, the qualities that make it suitable for animal respiration, the means of measuring its purity and of cleansing it when insalubrious, the procedures to combat the deleterious effects of putrid miasmas, the preparation of medicines of all kinds, the nature of poisons, animal, vegetable and mineral, their mode of operation, the most effective methods of controlling their harmful effects, the changes undergone by animal liquids and solids, under the influence of different diseases, the most effective measures to be taken to halt their progress and to alleviate the disorders which they have already produced; such are the important areas in which the physician can only attain an exact knowledge by the study of the principles of chemistry.

As already noted, in connection with Achille-Cléophas's earlier work with the chemist Thénard, chemistry is given pride of place in this speech. Homais, the opinionated village pharmacist in Madame Bovary, is a comically attenuated echo of this, Achille-Cléophas's favourite scientific theme.

Botany is useful to the physician by reason of the precious therapeutic remedies that it offers. Zoology alone can guide him to a complete knowledge of the human organism. The art of drawing, in describing various medical conditions, serves to capture details that words can only render imperfectly. It becomes indispensable in the case of organic disorders and deformities.

Since the physician needs to be acquainted with the whole range of the sciences, Monsieur Flaubert concludes that if he is required to be constantly observing and learning, then it is especially in the midst of learned societies that he can hope to acquire solid knowledge, that is to say he shall walk by the light of those who are extending the boundaries of the physical or the moral sciences.

These opportunities, which the Academy has put within his reach, inviting him into their midst, inspire in him an immense appreciation and an absolute loyalty towards this Company.[5]

That carefully encoded phrase, 'physical or moral sciences', points back in time to Cabanis and the radical materialism of the 1790s. There is some question as to whether the Academy was in business, after 1815, to 'extend the boundaries' or to police them. The evidence is inconclusive. Achille-Cléophas was actively engaged in the work of the Academy for at least the first five years of his membership. In that time he submitted eleven papers reviewing recent practical advances in medicine. Thereafter he withdrew and eventually resigned from the local Academy, though he remained an active member of other national networks, both medical and scientific.

For achille-cléophas, 1815 was a year of triumph. At the implausibly precocious and Napoleonic age of thirty-one, not only had he reached the summit of the medical profession, he had also been welcomed into the charmed circle that was Rouen Academy. Elsewhere, after Waterloo, the nation at large was experiencing conflicting emotions of chaotic intensity. The liberal, professional portion of that nation, those who had mostly done rather well out of the meritocratic years, were particularly disheartened by the prospect of monarchy restored. Adolphe Thiers, a rising young liberal journalist, voiced something of their prudently suppressed anger in his *History of the French Revolution* (1823): 'Frenchmen, we who have seen since then [i.e. 1815] our liberty stifled, our country invaded, our heroes shot or betraying their own glory, let us never forget those immortal days of liberty, greatness and hope!'[6]

Military defeat was consummated, in the summer of 1815, by a punitive second Treaty of Paris. That treaty restored Louis XVIII, confiscated choice portions of French territory and dictated a three-year military occupation to be paid for by the defeated. The delinquent revolutionary nation was now to be made to writhe and cringe, materially and morally, for its years of criminal exuberance. To supervise that delicately instructive process, more than one million foreign soldiers descended on the country for several years, like a horde of greedy houseguests, menacing and mocking their unhappy hosts.[7] In their wake, and equally resented, there came half a million émigré nobles, smiling victoriously at the restoration of birth and privilege.

Compulsory forgetting was the official state policy. Louis XVIII soon began to backdate his reign from the year 1795, the year that the previous heir to the throne had died, uncrowned, in a prison cell. In Rouen in November 1815, in accord with the strict new law on seditious items, the town council had zealously consigned to the flames on the Place Saint-Ouen a superb full-length Gros portrait of Napoleon.[8] It was not enough to hide the thing from view. It had to be ceremoniously destroyed. Conservation was 'a scandal that must be stopped. For it maintains the criminal hopes of the government's enemies.'[9] Could they have laid hands on the man himself, royalists would have had him strung up. Allowing the man to die of boredom on a remote and windswept island was a lamentable failure of nerve.

To assist the collective forgetting, sedition was now codified, formally and comprehensively. It could include anything that might 'corrupt the public spirit'.[10] In the public interest, thus loosely defined, the police set about removing from bookshops all works written and published during the Hundred Days. According to local police reports, all through the early 1820s, Rouen remained infected by 'seditious items'. The serious, persistent comedy of proscribed Napoleonic memories is best appreciated from a few prime local examples. At Christmas, for the festivities, the local confectioner, Daguillon, was found selling small statues of Bonaparte made in sugar and chocolate. In a local restaurant, a clandestine collection of twenty-four Napoleonic dinner plates was discovered. On a coach travelling from Paris to Rouen, the passengers were scandalised when a group of retired army officers openly displayed their Napoleonic tobacco boxes.[11]

Increasingly, through the 1820s, public servants, with Achille-Cléophas among their number, were required to be present at municipal ceremonies testifying to their political compliance. One such occasion occurred on 21 January 1822. It was the day of the first prescribed commemoration of the death of the Royal Martyr, Louis XVI, in 1793. Rouen, with its reputation for religious indifference, had been instructed to observe all ceremonies proper to a day of general mourning. Shops and theatres were to close. Ships in the harbour were to fly their flags at half-mast. The National Guard was to assemble in full uniform for a service in the cathedral. Representatives of the civil and military authorities were required to take part and fourteen local charities would make a special distribution to the poor.[12]

We may picture a reluctant but outwardly compliant Achille-Cléophas. On this day, his mood is complicated. As well as stifling his Voltairean sense of the ridiculous, he is remembering curiously parallel moments, at the Collège de Sens, back in the 1790s, when he was required as a schoolboy to attend the local festivals improvised by the theophilanthropists. He knows that the authorities are aware of his liberal political opinions. He also knows that they will leave him alone, on condition that he turns up in church when required and refrains from public expressions of dissent.

In the eyes of the church, this pragmatic state policy of active oblivion was not enough. Expiation was required. Crimes had been committed and forgiveness must be earned. To that end, the more zealous missionary factions organised spectacular public festivals that drew in thousands of spectators. It was intended to convert the rational citizens of the Republic, secular and anti-clerical, back into the loyal and pious subjects of the monarchy, Christian and Bourbon. Drawing on the local political geography, the missionaries led thousands of spectators in procession along the streets to the very place where, if condemned, they might once have faced the guillotine, twenty-five years earlier. Gathered around a large newly erected cross, adorned with the fleur-de-lys, there they listened to sermons, they sang canticles and they were led in prayer.[13] In Rouen in 1826, local hostility to this aggressive Catholic revival led to weeks of rioting. A touch of military intervention was required. The local archbishop, in fear for his life, went into hiding.

THE COUNTER-REVOLUTIONARY POLITICS of this troubled period weighed heavily on the secular liberal middle classes. Their freedom of expression, both collective and individual, was meticulously controlled. The poor, meanwhile, were beset by troubles of a different order.

The year 1816 was memorably hard, all across Europe, already exhausted from two decades of war. Early in April, there was an immense volcanic eruption in the Dutch East Indies. It was the largest eruption for over one thousand years. Mount Tambora poured so much ash into the atmosphere that average summer temperatures in France fell by three degrees centigrade. The sun hazed over, the plants died, the harvest failed and the food riots began. The year 1816 was the last great subsistence crisis in Western Europe.

In the countryside around Rouen, gangs of beggars and vagabonds roamed about at night, extracting charitable donations of food from the larder of any farmer. In the city, crowds attacked baker's shops. Soldiers were brought in to restore order. The prefect observed: 'We cannot hide the fact that there is unrest and ill-will everywhere, and that all the markets where we do not deploy strong forces will be the scene of disorder and crime.' The prefect appealed to the 'charitable souls of this town' to contribute to a special fund to subsidise the price of bread to the poor. In mid-June the price of bread spiked at 0.94 francs per kilo, three times the ordinary subsistence level. The town council criticised charities. Paupers don't like the third-rate charity bread. They have seen it being swapped for white bread, for cake and for strong liquor. There followed much loose bourgeois talk of the feckless poor: the vagabonds, the fakers, the fugitives, the jailbirds, the women and children who beg for a living, the imprudent, those who drink their wages away.[14]

Working in the Hôtel-Dieu, Achille-Cléophas was well placed to observe how all these modern miseries were written upon the bodies of his patients. It was surely not a comfortable position, morally or professionally. On the one hand, it was not his job to campaign on behalf of the wretched of the Earth. To do so would obviously antagonise all those who, in a spirit of Christian charity, administered the Hôtel-Dieu. On the other hand, Achille-Cléophas was required to deal with the casualties of urbanisation, patient by patient. He knew that he must confine himself to the immediate task. He would do the surgery. The nuns could do the spiritual welfare. The radicals, if there were still any out there, could do the liberty and the equality.

By the year 1815, Rouen's social problem had been public knowledge for at least ten years. In 1804 the Municipal Council deplored the fact that 'of all manufacturing towns, Rouen is perhaps the one where the workers have the worst housing'.[15] For the next forty years, very little was going to change. In spite of a high mortality rate, the population of the city grew from 80,000 to 100,000. The newcomers were pulled in year after year from the villages by the prospect of high wages in the textile mills and by the greater everyday liberty of city life.

Infant mortality in Rouen was exceptionally high. One third of newborn infants died in the first year of life. In a hungry winter, babies were regularly found abandoned in church doorways. There had always been foundlings and the church had always taken them in. But it was the rising number of foundlings that caused concern. In January 1813, in an effort to reduce mortality, an ingeniously screened wooden turntable was installed in the door of the local hospice. Outside in the street, the baby was placed on the turntable. Rotating it by half a turn, the baby was conveyed safely inside. The anonymity of the parent and the life of the baby were both preserved. If you hoped to come back for your baby in future years, it was the custom to leave one half of a small distinctive scrap of printed fabric tied to the wrist or the ankle. When you returned ten years later with your identical scrap, you could reclaim your child.[16]

Urbanisation exacerbated all those ills that we now regard as 'public health problems'. Acknowledging a collective responsibility for dealing with the miscellaneous filth that besets everyday life, the phrase 'public health' encapsulates a debate that could not be resolved within the lifetime of Achille-Cléophas. There was, to put it simply, an ideological impasse. As a recent historian has argued: 'Their science rendered public a dis-heartening record of poverty, sickness and early death. Their eyes beheld the full spectrum of human degradation. Their social convictions told them […] the state could do nothing because it should do nothing.'[17]

The dismal science of political economy said that state intervention was not the correct response to current problems. Economic salvation must remain an individual matter. In some quarters, debauchery and the sloth of the workers was thought to be the most frequent cause of their destitution,[18] though more soberly enlightened views were emerging. This is Villermé, the public health expert, reporting on social conditions in Rouen in the 1830s:

> When in work, with wages at their ordinary level, with bread at a moderate price, a couple can live within their joint income if they have no children. With one child there is already little to spare. With two or three children it is impossible to live within the household income. The family will be obliged to depend on charity until the children reach a working age.[19]

Meanwhile, in the words of a report published in Rouen in 1842: 'Pauperism is making rapid and fearsome progress. In a society ever more enlightened, ever more policed, ever more prosperous, even as the material means of comfort and happiness increase, so too does misery, hideous and repulsive misery, increase and multiply.'[20] By the late 1830s, it was obvious that several generations of urban poverty had produced adults who were too feeble for the army. The response came in 1841, with a law limiting child labour.[21]

For a faintly macabre postscript to the social question, we may contemplate, within the same frame, the first and last moments of a life lived in the shadow of this same social question. On the first page, the discarded baby is laid upon the turntable at the door of the convent. On the last page, the condemned man, is strapped down, in the prison yard, beneath the great blade that will so humanely see him off.

Achille-Cléophas had a legitimate professional interest in this particular terminal social fact. To teach anatomy, he needed fresh corpses. In 1819, he wrote the following letter to the Administration concerning the supply of suitable medical material from the local prison:

> The Director will supply me with all the means at his command to increase and to facilitate our dissections to maintain both the propriety and the salubrity in our laboratories. One thing is often lacking when we wish to demonstrate how anatomy contributes to surgical operations: cadavers that are neither corrupted nor emaciated by disease, nor already spoilt by one or two days that have elapsed since the moment of death. Only executions can meet our requirements and often we are unable to obtain them. On the other hand, nothing could be more beneficial than having possession of these individuals whose almost living organs still have the volume and the density of the organs of men in good health, and upon which operations would best resemble those which the students are required to perform upon our patients.[22]

14

Two Nations

Uninterrupted disturbance of all social conditions, everlasting uncertainty and agitation […] a society that has conjured up such gigantic means of production and exchange, is like the sorcerer, who is no longer able to control the powers of the nether world whom he has called up by his spells.

— KARL MARX, *The Communist Manifesto* (1848)

A S A PUBLIC SERVANT, as well as an eminent member of one of the liberal professions, Achille-Cléophas was by now, in the early 1820s, a significant presence in the bourgeois public sphere; though he would not have recognised that precise phrase, for it belongs to a later age. The public sphere, briskly defined, is that social space in which informed critical conversation can flourish. The Rouen Academy, an institution that we have already visited, was one such place. The local newspapers of the day were another such.

The *Journal de Rouen* is of particular interest. In the 1820s it spoke out, emphatically and consistently, on behalf of those who, like Achille-Cléophas, were the reluctant but compliant subjects of the restored House of Bourbon. Voltairean and Saint-Simonian in outlook, it had been founded in the 1780s by a friend of Diderot. Now a platform for the contemporary liberal values of class unity around the theme of useful work, the *Journal de Rouen* was finely tuned to the material interests and the cultural aspirations of a prosperous modernising local elite. By 1846 it had built a circulation of three thousand.[1]

In an editorial from 25 January 1831, that readership is succinctly defined as 'men who acknowledge no other entitlement than that of hard work, no other superiority than that of enlightenment and intelligence, no other title to social advantage than that which is earned by service to society as a whole.' These are the men who are the truly useful, as opposed to 'men who consider that power and influence and prosperity are the exclusive domain of the few, a set of privileges existing by virtue of a kind of mysterious legitimacy.' From everything we know about his history, we can say that Achille-Cléophas fits that profile. He would have read the *Journal de Rouen* and, as one of the local elite, he may well have known the editor.[2]

Explicit evidence, both for Achille-Cléophas's opinions and for his intelligent caution in expressing them, is contained in a security report, compiled in 1824 by an official in the local prefecture, for transmission to the Ministry of the Interior in Paris. The relevant portion reads as follows: 'This doctor's political opinions are liberal, but he has never been seen in the role of advocate. His speeches on the contrary indicate wisdom and moderation, and his behaviour is such that even those who do not share his principles generally accord him their confidence.'[3]

Examining the pages of the *Journal de Rouen*, we may map, with some probability, the themes of unconstrained conversation among Achille-Cléophas and his circle. I have chosen the early months of 1822 as the focus for this conjectural group portrait.

IN JANUARY, revived after a long gap in publication, the *Journal* invited citizens to send in their poems and letters, the 'fruits of their leisure'. That excellent phrase evokes precisely the local civic culture of the hour: amateur, leisured and literate and predominantly masculine; the readers are liberals in the early sense of that word and they are aware of the the poor as distant objects of compassion. The *Journal* reported a New Year speech by the archbishop of Rouen blessing the chapel of the local orphanage, praising the church's social mission and the pious intentions of its benefactors. The archbishop foretells a world in which 'Misery will be stripped of it rags and the unfortunate will be made forever happy.' Meanwhile, on the fifteenth of the month there is a civic funeral procession for a local judge. In that procession, a hundred paupers each carry a loaf of bread and a candle.

According to a recent law, this year on 21 January there is to be an official commemoration of the death of Louis XVI the Royal Martyr.

General mourning is decreed. The *Journal* reports the debate in the chamber of deputies, bitterly contesting the laws imposing fines for insulting religion, monarchy and the state. It is proving difficult to establish constitutional government. Historic recrimination, going back to 1789, is the order of the day. A characteristic exchange between legitimists and liberals includes the following: 'It should come as no surprise that men raised in the school of revolution and usurpation should have no understanding of the doctrine of fidelity.' This provokes what the *Journal* calls 'violent murmurings on the left.'

On 9 February, the *Journal* announced official approval for a school of medicine based in Rouen hospitals. Henceforth, from the first day of January until the first day of May, every morning at ten o'clock in the Hôtel-Dieu, Achille-Cléophas Flaubert will give courses in anatomy and physiology. On Mondays, Wednesdays and Fridays at eleven in the morning, Achille-Cléophas will be running a clinic for outpatients.

For all its modernity, Rouen had preserved some older urban traditions. On 15 February the *Journal* reported a day of carnival celebrations. The illustrious variety artist Gringalet was seen in costume at the head of a glorious cavalcade, with a decorated float of maskers that passed through all quarters of the city accompanied by large crowds. Molière played at the theatre that same evening, followed by a splendid masked ball. The *Journal* drew the moral: 'Everywhere we observed that contentment that is solely the result of the current happy state of peace and of the prosperity of our commerce.'

In March, from a somewhat different Catholic and royalist perspective, the vicar general called the blessing of St Louis on the city. Evidently the lines of political difference were still very tightly drawn. It may be a symptom of the same mood that when the Royal Academy announced the theme of its annual essay prize it proposed a splendidly anodyne topic in local history: the administrative structures of medieval Normandy.

In the month of May, two further announcements catch the eye. The first item reveals the enduring complexity of the medical world, in which science and superstition still coexist. In a brief paragraph, Dr Lusardi, honorary oculist to the Duchess of Parma, announces his presence in the city of Rouen and he invites the afflicted to attend him at the Hôtel de France. In the course of the next few weeks the *Journal* publishes a list of those whom he has so miraculously cured, suggesting that Dr Lusardi ought to be paid from the public purse to minister to the poor. The second item points into the future. A thirty-horsepower one-hundred-foot-long iron steamboat, the *Aaron Mamby*, made in Birmingham, has docked in Rouen en route to Paris. The *Aaron Mamby's* paddle wheel, a new design, more compact and more efficient, is exciting great public curiosity.

IN 1821, THE YEAR OF GUSTAVE'S BIRTH, Achille-Cléophas consummated the first phase of his professional success with the purchase of a house in the country. The property cost 52,000 francs. Husband and wife shared the cost equally. Her money no doubt gave her voice a distinctive authority in the marital conversation. Equally, that same money gave Achille-Cléophas a certain careless energy in his dealings with the world. On the most recent electoral register he had declared an annual rental income from property of 1,340 francs, sufficient to qualify for a vote under the restricted property franchise of the day.

In 1821 he was on the threshold of the most fulfilling chapter of his life. He was now thirty-seven years old, at the height of his powers, widely esteemed and plentifully rewarded. Since becoming a member of the local Academy in 1815, he had presented eleven papers. This suggests that he was, for the moment at least, securely integrated into the elite. Perhaps he might begin to look beyond local horizons. Ambitious thoughts were privately encouraged when he was mentioned, in a Parisian almanac for 1825, as 'one of the foremost doctors in France'.[4]

He had now been married for nine years and had fathered four children. Two of those children had survived and two had died in the first year of life. There would eventually be two more births, and one more infant death. Such high levels of infant mortality were a lamentable fact of urban life, even among the elite. But what can we say of the experience of bereavement at that time and in that place? In the mind of a man such as Achille-Cléophas, a disciple of Voltaire and Bichat, educated in the critical materialist philosophy of his generation, the cult of the dear departed could be neither confessed or sustained.

The critical materialist's wife, an orphan of the Revolution raised in a convent, may well have felt differently. It was not unusual at this time, in this social class, for husband and wife to agree to differ in matters of religion. Religious indifference, shading into anti-clericalism, was the province of men, especially men of education and energy. Orthodox

religious faith was for women. It was an endearing, decorative, poeti-
cal thing; more to the point, it kept women in line. Caroline Fleuriot
evidently brought her Catholic faith into her early married life. In the
1830s she was *dame patronesse* of a local convent school for orphans.[5]
That was a laudable gesture of reparation for all that she herself had lost
as a child. Her faith, at least in its outward philanthropic expression,
endured until the late 1840s. At that point, according to her younger son
Gustave, after the deaths of her husband and her daughter, she 'suddenly
became an atheist'.[6]

For the moment, such painful events were still far away in the future.
The next two children, Gustave (1821) and Caroline (1824), would both
survive into adulthood. With three children, two sons and a daughter,
the now completed family could begin to enjoy their new house in the
country. An hour's journey by carriage from the Hôtel-Dieu, this was a
modest, handsome property standing on the hillside just above the village of Déville. Set fifty metres back from the road and sheltered by a
double row of elm trees, the house had a wide terrace and gardens that
looked out across the fields and down into the valley below. The main
house came with a cluster of adjacent buildings, a small farm with a cider
press, a stable-block and a barn. Discreetly delighted by the magnitude
of his worldly success, Achille-Cléophas purchased a bust of Hippocrates
and put it on display in a niche just above the front door. Evidently the
entrepreneurs of the new scientific medicine had not rejected their comfortably remote ancestors.

This Déville house, with the eventual addition of left and right wings,
remained in the family's possession for twenty-odd years, all through
Gustave Flaubert's childhood. Here in the garden, at the age of ten, he
organised the local children into a small army of National Guards.[7] It was
a pleasant refuge, a world away from the family's cramped and melancholy
quarters in the Hôtel-Dieu. Even so, it was not entirely insulated from
the crude and encroaching powers of the industrial nineteenth century.
When you were standing under the trees in the garden at Déville, you
could hear the sound of a factory steam-engine in the next valley. In the
distance, just beyond the village and the church tower, you could see a
cluster of factory chimneys, a curious and portentous addition to the
landscape.

The view from the garden of the new house was still pleasantly and
predominantly rural. But Déville, the village down in the valley, was no

agricultural Arcadia. It was an industrial zone and it had been so for several centuries. The swift-flowing local river, the Cailly, a tributary of the Seine, was perfect for water power. Paper mills had arrived on the banks of the river in the sixteenth century. One of the earliest cotton mills had been built there in the 1760s. Steam power, with its more intrusive chimneys, noise and smoke was already well established in the valley by the time of the Flaubert family's arrival in 1821. When Achille-Cléophas eventually sold the Déville property in 1844, it was because the new railway line was about to take a large slice out of his garden.

THE DYNAMIC TEXTILE SECTOR of the new industrial order ran on steam power, gaslight and unskilled labour. In Rouen, as elsewhere, that labour force was mostly youthful, illiterate and chronically exhausted. Mademoiselle Berthe Bovary, daughter of Charles and Emma, on the last page of the novel remembered principally for the death of her mother, is finally orphaned and sent, by her impoverished aunt, to work in a cotton factory. It's a curious, unobtrusive detail, placed out at the very edge of the social vision of that novel. For a child from a middle-class family to find herself working in cotton factory was a fate so dark that it could not be imagined in any detail. Imaginatively invisible and politically ignored, early nineteenth-century factory work was undoubtedly a form of slow death, at least until the laws of the late 1840s began to reform and regulate the labour market, mitigating some of the more extreme forms of exploitation.

In the city of Rouen, all through the hard angry years from 1815 until around 1845, much of the incidental human damage caused by this exceptionally voracious process found its way to the gates of the Hôtel-Dieu. There, the surgical cases became the clinical responsibility of the physicians working under the direction of Achille-Cléophas. In his professional capacity, he was aware of the connection between public health and general living conditions. It was obvious to anyone not blinded by self-interest.

In a jointly authored document from the year 1834, Achille-Cléophas and his senior colleague, Dr Hellis, set out their decorously constrained understanding of the contemporary social question. They are describing both the patients in the Hôtel-Dieu and the inmates of the associated hospice-asylum:

A hospital dedicated to the indigent of a large city will feel the effects of everything that bears upon the lives of the unfortunate. The high cost of bread, workers being laid off, the rigours of winter, these things push a large number of people into a state of need. Their refuge is the hospital. We cannot refuse admission to those who are perishing from the cold, those who are destitute, or those who find that, for whatever reason, the infirmities to which they are subject have become momentarily worse. The needy, their numbers greatly increased every winter, arriving in great waves during any public disaster, the needy are not sick. Bread and shelter is all they ask, until the better weather allows them to find work.[8]

Looking through the manuscript collection of Achille-Cléophas's case histories from the years 1818–22, we can enter into the human detail of that larger urban social history. From among the five hundred cases briefly recorded, I have chosen a handful of representative individuals. Their presenting problems include chronic ailments caused by poor housing, industrial accidents caused by a moment's inattention at work and lingering psychological problems caused by recent experiences on the battlefield. I have woven commentary and explanation into the body of the case history. In these laconic matter-of-fact texts, the local condition of the working class comes into focus with a lucidly excruciating particularity.

Ferdinand Dubos, admitted to the Hôtel-Dieu on 19 June 1819 (one of the hungriest months of the year). The boy is eight and half years old. He has worked in a textile factory, probably since the age of eight, and he has a strong constitution. (It was not unusual, in these unregulated years, to find children of this age working in textile factories. One of the first generation of French public health experts, when he visited a Rouen cotton-spinning factory in the year 1831, found that one in three of the workforce was under the age of fifteen. In that same factory, one in ten was under the age of ten.)[9]

With his left hand Ferdinand Dubos was turning the handle on a big wheel. To help his balance, he had his right arm stretched out straight. The right arm was caught between the spokes of the big wheel as it turned. The boy was dragged into the machinery, fracturing the lower portion of the arm. It bled copiously in two places where the bone had been displaced. Within two hours of the accident, a surgeon 'reduced' the fracture, applied a bandage and sent the boy to the Hôtel-Dieu. There, they remove the bandage in order to establish the precise nature of the fracture. They stop the bleeding and then bind the arm in a splint. The pulse was strong and regular. The boy yawned a great deal and was not hungry. He was discharged after several days.[10]

Aimable Vassé, from Rouen, boy aged fourteen, machinist, contracted a head cold six months ago, quite severe, now cured. The eyes were oozing and for the last three days have become inflamed due to the irritation caused by small particles of cotton waste.[11] (Dr Hellis, one of Achille-Cléophas's colleagues, calculated in 1826 that the machinist spinning cotton on the jenny-mule was inhaling around 300g of cotton waste every day, causing chronic lung disease as well as eye infections.)

Marie d'Amour, aged sixteen, living in Rouen, admitted to the Hôtel-Dieu on 14 February 1819 with a chronic opthalmia (inflammation of the eye). This young woman is not yet menstruating and lives in damp conditions; she has been subject to this opthalmia for about the last five years and has been to the hospital several times, where she was cured with vesicatories to the neck and leeches on the eyelids, but almost as soon as she returned home the condition recurred with greater intensity.[12]

Théodore Giffosse, aged nineteen, fairly strong constitution, dye worker exposed alternatively to humidity and then great heat, about a week ago experienced pains in his joints. He continued working, but the pains were so intense that he was obliged to leave work and take some rest. Resting for several days at home he experienced no relief; he was admitted to the Hôtel-Dieu on 30 March.[13]

Augustin l'Aîné, aged nineteen, dye worker, fairly strong constitution, had a fall on 11 March 1820; his right leg went into a vat of boiling dye. Extricated, the leg was red but not swollen. He was immediately conveyed home where he was advised to apply a compress of vinegar and salt water to his leg. He was admitted that same evening to the Hôtel-Dieu, the whole leg then swollen, red and painful.[14]

Paul Dominique Bigault, aged twenty-three, from Rouen, a weaver, admitted 28 January 1819, complains he cannot distinguish objects at twenty paces; this problem appears to be the consequence of a moment of great terror four years ago when this young man saw pieces of dead bodies on a battlefield. Since that time, his sight has grown progressively weaker.[15]

Robert Jean, textile worker, aged twenty-five, living in Déville, on the seventh of this month having gone into the forest at four in the morning was surprised by a gamekeeper who fired upon him at a distance of about six paces with a shotgun hitting the right side of the head. Two pieces of shot went into the right eye, one split the upper eyelid, the other cut into the sclerotic membrane. The patient was admitted on 8 March with the following: swollen face, intelligence confused, rapid pulse, edges of the two eye-sockets inflamed, the right eye presenting the two incisions.[16]

The next case history illustrates an industrial injury of the slow chronic variety. The injury is caused by repetitive work on the jenny-mule, one of the giant new machines for spinning cotton, machines that depended on the strength and brute force of the operator, pushing forward and pulling back the heavy frame, four times a minute, for hour after hour.

Bongos, aged twenty-eight, a fairly good constitution, a machinist at Rouen, having worked for ten years as a sailor, enduring frequent atmospheric insults without ever having been diagnosed with any serious disease; changing profession, he began to work on the jenny-mule, a type of work that he has followed for the last five years. About two years ago, Bongos felt rheumatic pain in the area of the kidneys, the stomach, the left shoulder-joints and the right knee-joint. The pain varied according to temperature changes, often very intense; in the winter, they diminished with the return of spring and became almost zero in summer. All these pains having moved away from their primary site, about six weeks ago they seemed to focus around the femoro-tiborial joint and towards the beginning of April 1819, the pains having increased to a higher level of intensity without swelling, the patient came to consult Mr Flaubert, who prescribed the application of six leeches every five days, emollient poultices and rest. The latter having not been observed, Bongos returned as usual to working at the jenny-mule. He soon saw the intensity of his pain increase and his condition degenerate to a cold tumour, a change that decided him to enter the Hôtel-Dieu on 26 April 1819, presenting with a swelling of the right knee joint, pain sometimes quite intense felt especially in the internal part of the joint. Above the kneecap, there is a tumour about two inches in size full of lymphatic fluid; 26 April, application of emollient poultices; 27 April, prescribed four scarifying cups. Still a very serious condition and very common example of a rheumatic disease in the first stages and which, having attached itself to a joint, has caused a tumour. During this observation the habitual failure of the sick to take rest and conditions often incurable resulting from this disobedience was also noted. The patient was discharged unhealed in the first days of June.[17]

Working the machines in the textile factories was dangerous. The work often required the operator to go inside the machine to clean or to adjust it. The last of these specimen case histories concerns one such incident.

Catherine Niel, aged forty-four, machinist, fairly good constitution, living in Rouen, rue St Hilaire, had her head caught in a machine on 23 October 1822. She was admitted the same day, presenting the following symptoms: fainting, loss of consciousness, speech impaired, general debility, severe pains in the head, copious loss of blood through the nose and the ears, blood seeping from the right eyelid and from the mouth. A short time after her arrival she vomited a bloody liquid mixed with food.[18]

AFTER THESE INDIVIDUAL HISTORIES, it may be time to enlarge the frame. We shall consider three contending descriptions of this darkening urban landscape, descriptions written by three witnesses who, for different reasons, made it their business to understand, to manage or simply to document the changes that were taking place in the city they knew. They were respectively an industrialist, a physician and a factory worker.

In the wake of the July Revolution of 1830, many who had previously been excluded from public life were now advanced to positions of power. Accordingly, the royalist mayor of Rouen, the marquis de Martainville, was replaced by a man more in tune with the new regime. Henri Barbet was an industrialist, a liberal grandee and a man with a strongly conservative social agenda. Barbet's father had amassed a fortune in textiles in the 1790s, manufacturing *indiennes*, the bright machine-printed fabrics that were made into women's skirts, men's cravats and waistcoats. Barbet, co-owner of Barbet Frères, was a model of vigorous, second-generation diversification. He had a group of factories, as well as interests in banking and – eventually – in railway construction. He was also a man with a simple answer to the Social Question.

Barbet served as mayor of Rouen for seventeen years, from 1830. His proudest achievement, for he found the time to write it up, lay in cleansing Rouen of the six hundred idle paupers, men, women and children, who lived by begging. Barbet's campaign and the thinking behind it were much celebrated. It was even known as the *système Barbet* and it furnished an ideal topic for educated dinner-table conversation, both frivolous and compassionate.

In the course of ten years, Barbet cleansed the streets. This is how he described the process in an open letter to a politician colleague, published in 1841:

> In this town where one used to find a beggar on every street, on every promenade, in the doorways of churches and shops; in this town where the eye was assailed by the sight of hideous, spurious sores eagerly displayed to elicit the compassion of the passer-by; in this same town where gangs of beggars, a hundred strong, would congregate at certain houses on certain days to ask for alms from those who gave regularly and indiscriminately; in this same town today one scarcely ever comes across even one furtive beggar, and he can be immediately arrested, thanks to the tireless vigilance of the police.[19]

One began with a proper survey of the problem, for it was alarmingly deep-rooted. It soon emerged that there were around six hundred persistent beggars in the city. Many were well established on their patch. Four or five generations of the same family had occupied the same church door, or the same street corner. They regarded their spot as an item of property, something to pass on, to sell or to hire out, if an heir were lacking. This feature of the street culture, Barbet finds scandalous and fascinating. It seems that even the destitute have this property instinct, perverted though it appears to be.

The next step is to classify. It is established that 20 per cent are men, 20 per cent are children and 60 per cent are women. Fifteen per cent are crippled, some with leg ulcers, some with amputations, some simply from old age. The elderly and infirm are no more than 5 per cent. Many of those displaying their sores are faking. Most of these beggars are mere idlers. Idle ever since childhood. The exceptions, the genuinely destitute, are proudly reluctant to beg on the streets. They knock on the doors of certain private houses, where they know they will be kindly received. They make very little, compared to their professional rivals who can easily clear three or four francs a day, a sum that is significantly more than a day's wages for an adult male factory worker. Indeed, some of the professionals have accumulated thousands of francs in secret savings.

Barbet's scheme of 'social protection' was a masterly blend of compulsion and compassion. Genuine cripples were accommodated in local charity hospitals. The workhouses were closed. Women and children swept the streets and the men did road mending. All were told that it was against the law to beg. To show that this was serious, a few veteran idlers were arrested and imprisoned overnight. Wages on the work scheme were kept low, so as not to draw labour away from the factories. The local churches and the local courts both supported Barbet's campaign. Indeed the archbishop insisted that this humane and prudent scheme in no way conflicted with the traditional Christian duty of charity towards the poor. The campaign produced a nice array of miracles: incurable sores disappeared, the blind recovered their sight and cripples rose to their feet, throwing down the crutches adopted twenty years ago.

In Part 3 of *Madame Bovary*, there is a lunatic blind beggar who haunts the woods on the road between the village of Yonville and the city of Rouen. He is a disconcertingly imagined version of the creatures that were, in the 1830s, the object of *le système Barbet*.

> A mass of rags covered his shoulders, and a squashed beaver hat, bent down into the shape of a bowl, concealed his face; but, when he took it off, he exposed, instead of eyelids, two yawning bloodstained holes. The flesh was tattered into scarlet strips; and fluid was trickling out, congealing into green crusts that reached down to his nose, with black nostrils that kept sniffing convulsively. Whenever he spoke, he threw back his head with an idiot laugh; – then his blue eyes, rolling convulsively, would graze the edges of the open sores, near both his temples.[20]

Gustave Flaubert wants to make us see, to make us look, closely and compassionately, at the thing from which we habitually turn away. He wants to correct our vision, by this precise and humane notation of the conventionally disgusting. In this, he is the worthy heir of the enlightened physician.

On the other hand Monsieur Homais, the village pharmacist, conducts a Barbet-style campaign against this same blind beggar. At one point, Homais exclaims: 'I cannot understand why it is that the authorities still tolerate such scandalous activities. Those wretched people ought to be locked away and made to do some work.'[21] Failing to cure the blind man with one of his ointments, Homais 'trained his guns on him in a campaign that revealed the depth of his intelligence and the malevolence of his vanity.'[22] He has the man incarcerated, then condemned to perpetual confinement in an asylum. By the end of the novel, Homais is in control of everything. The final sentences of the novel record his triumph: 'He is doing infernally well; the authorities handle him carefully and public opinion is on his side. He has just received the Legion of Honour.'[23]

BARBET, THE LOCAL INDUSTRIALIST, administered his city from behind a large desk in a well-appointed office. Dr Eugène Hellis, as a physician trained in the new social medicine, knew that same city in the raw. In his mind, it was the smell of a damp overcrowded house, with the sound of coughing coming from above. In his notebook, it was annual statistics of infant mortality.

Hellis was ten years younger than Achille-Cléophas, a devout Catholic, a good friend of the archbishop and a bachelor with a private income and a weekly salon. Hellis and Achille-Cléophas could have been designed to antagonise one another. Hellis stood for everything that was detestable about the Restoration. Even more challengingly, he was of the rising generation, one of those who thought in a new way about the scope of medicine.

In 1818, in a public session of the Academy, Achille-Cléophas had seriously impugned Hellis's clinical competence and his professional honesty. Here was mediocrity incarnate. Nonetheless, Hellis was appointed as deputy to the chief of the medical division at the Hôtel-Dieu in 1820. He was only twenty-six years old and he was climbing the ladder even more rapidly than Achille-Cléophas had done. A few years later, in a letter to the Commission, Achille-Cléophas blocked their proposal to promote Hellis as his new deputy. He explained to them that he could not work with a man who 'three years ago could not answer the simplest question', a man whose skills in surgery had faded from lack of practice.

Whatever his personal qualities, Hellis was conspicuously diligent. His published work from the 1820s chronicles the various material conditions that determined public health. He looks beyond the walls of the Hôtel-Dieu and beyond the clinical profile of the individual patient. Attuned to the progressive medical thinking of the day, his work is distinctively if naively statistical, geographical and meteorological. He makes hundreds of observations and he tabulates them. But Hellis is also moved by an active humanitarian compassion for the plight of urban poor. This informed sympathy has its roots in the religious duty of charity.

Predictably, such sympathy was tempered by worldly self-interest. In 1826, when Hellis published his book on conditions in Rouen, he did not include any of the material he had put together on the contentious topic of chronic diseases among workers in the textile industry. Publishing it might have displeased one of the overlords who served on the Commission that ran the Hôtel-Dieu where Hellis was employed. That material did not emerge until 1998, when a local historian discovered the complete manuscript.

In Hellis's published account, Rouen is 'a city equally renowned for its antiquity, its drab condition and its impure air.'[24] The eastern portion of the town, previously marshy, has been drained, filled in and converted into a parade ground for the splendid new barracks. Yet this has scarcely improved the worst parts of the city. The houses are too close together. They are chronically damp. The streets are crooked, narrow and squalid. The main street is damp and stinking from the market debris.

By the 1820s three quarters of the local workforce were engaged in the textile industry. The worst health risks were in the cotton factories. While processing the raw cotton fibres an individual worker could inhale 300g–400g of dust every day. 'I find it hard to believe', wrote Hellis, 'that any women could keep up this kind of work for several years without damaging even the strongest chest. Their faces, yellow, colourless, or livid, their emaciation, their continuous coughing, the colour of their cheeks, a sure sign of damaged lungs, all clearly indicate the fate which lies in wait for them.' The medical profession called it *adynamism*, a state of physiological exhaustion. It was notoriously common among the textile workers of Rouen.[25]

WHATEVER THEIR DIFFERENCES, Barbet, Hellis and Achille-Cléophas all moved in the upper world of monogrammed linen, bespoke tailoring and vintage wines. The testimony of our third witness comes from a parallel world, from the factory floor.

Charles Noiret was a working-class autodidact, the child of illiterate rural linen-weavers who moved to Rouen in the late 1790s to work in the new textile factories. Exceptionally intelligent, curious and determined, Noiret attended one of the free schools recently set up in the city. He entered the historical record in 1832, when he was awarded a silver medal by a local philanthropic society for improvements to the weaving process.

These improvements he had devised and donated, for the public good, without claiming the inventor's royalties to which he was legally entitled.

Encouraged by this recognition, Noiret submitted, to the society that gave him the medal, a series of critical essays on the great social questions of the day. When none of his essays was published in the official bulletin, Noiret found an ally in the newly appointed radical young editor of the local newspaper, the *Journal de Rouen*. Voice of the progressive liberal opposition, anti-clerical and Saint-Simonian, the *Journal de Rouen* was intent on unsettling the new mayor, that eminent plutocrat Barbet. Noiret was clearly the man for the job. He was amusingly disrespectful, he was in touch with working-class experience and he could write fluently.

Here he is, in full flight, on the subject of the vexations endured by patients on the wards of the Hôtel-Dieu.

> Thinking about the hospital, I would like to know if it is for saving their souls or for getting them back to health, that the poor go there when they are sick; if it is to save their souls then they ought to get rid of the kitchen, the pharmacy, the doctors and the surgeons and even the beds, because you don't need any of that stuff to get to paradise; but if it is to bring them back to health then they really ought to do something about the religious business, which disturbs the peace and hinders the recovery of the sick. Every day, first thing in the morning, a man goes through the wards ringing a great big bell and shouting at the top of his voice to announce the mass. This is a sudden rude awakening for the sick; it affects their morale and deprives them of the sleep that they often miss in the night. In the wards where mass is said there is an enormous racket. From three in the morning in winter there is sweeping and polishing and benches and chairs being moved; you can't hear yourself think; all this housework not only stops the sick from sleeping, it annoys them. Finally, when it is time for mass, the sick are invited along; it is true that they are not forced into it, but the nuns nag them so much that in the end they get out of bed, set off for paradise and catch a fever on the way. And while I'm on the subject I would like to ask the medical gentlemen at the Hôtel-Dieu if they would stop their students from blocking the corridors on visit days and scandalising people, especially the women, by improper suggestions and rude songs.[26]

In 1836 then, at the age of thirty-four, after twenty years on the weaving machines, Noiret published locally a book of one hundred pages, entitled *Mémoires d'un ouvrier rouennais*. In substance, and in ambition, this was the very first publication of its kind. Noiret's aim, as advertised on the first page, is not autobiographical. It is, he says, to 'denounce abuses so as to put an end to them'. In that fighting spirit, the book begins with a briskly but vulnerably polemical account of the local shift from artisan to industrial production, with loss of quality in the product, loss of dignity in the worker and fraudulent petty practices among the owners.

More original and more sombre, because grounded in the detail of the author's own experiences, is the subsequent portrait of his own section of the workforce, the weavers. Framed as a response to an industrial inquiry promoted by a leftist journal in Paris, it stands as a fine essay in what will later be called history from below. Noiret's generation of weavers, with their family memories of lost artisan liberties, found themselves subject to the disciplines of de-skilled factory labour and the destructive caprices of the trade cycle. They were waking to a form of class-consciousness. Noiret's memoir voices this befuddled ethical moment of awakening, with its nostalgia, its indignation, its denunciation of abuses and its utopian schemes of regeneration.

The central portion of Noiret's text is structured as a dialogue, with brief questions and extended answers. The two 'speakers' are not named or individualised. We are at an imaginary public inquiry into social conditions. We are getting at the truth, piece by piece, by means of sober testimony, as if we were in a courtroom. The form of the text reproduces the emergent class alliance between the educated worker and that familiar elusive figure, the Friend of the People. The friend is a lawyer, or a journalist or a politician, or some combination of the three; the friend is the agent of a process that is empowering and constraining in equal measure. Noiret's hybrid form of memoir-inquiry testifies to the difficulty of combining subjective and objective visions of the occulted world of manual labour. It was still too soon, in 1836, for a realist narrative.

The final magisterial word on the social question shall come from high in the clouds. Under the headword *Hygiène (Moderne)*, the 1818 edition of the *Dictionary of Medical Sciences* includes the following passage:

O people of the cities, it is for you that such sacrifices have been made! And it is for you that the solicitude of governments strives to protect you from all harmful influences; it is for you above all that the public highways have been cleaned; it is for you that magnificent and salubrious promenades have been built; for you that we have removed from beneath your eyes those deep chambers where your mortal remains will one day decay! It is for you that artistically designed sewers have been built, places more habitable than the hovels of the poor, and for you that conduits have been constructed at great expense to bring forth clean water […] it is truly for you that public hygiene is studied and practiced! Everything encourages us to hope that these exceptional exertions will reach out to those quarters where misery cries out, where industry, strenuous and weary, takes shelter, and is not confined to those places where opulence and ease reside. One day we shall no longer see, alongside the sumptuous edifices of an opulent city, the obscenity of a filthy river […] that flows through the sanctuaries of the indigent.[27]

A sudden and magnificent peroration, in the midst of a sober dictionary entry, this passage captures perfectly both the Enlightenment aspiration to perfectibility and its apparently incurable early nineteenth-century disappointment. Achille-Cléophas had *The Dictionary of Medical Sciences* in his personal library; the passage in question was written by his influential Parisian mentor, Jean-Noël Hallé. We can be confident that Achille-Cléophas would have read it. By contrast, in Charles Bovary's consulting room, we discover evidence of a man neglecting his professional development: 'The volumes of *The Dictionary of Medical Sciences*, uncut, but with their bindings damaged from being bought and sold so frequently, were the sole adornment of the six shelves of the pinewood bookcase.'[28]

15

Fear and Trembling

This scourge, if it had come upon us in an age of religion [...] would have left behind a vivid picture. Imagine a black flag flying from the towers of Notre Dame, the cannon firing single shots now and again, to warn the thoughtless traveller to turn back; a ring of troops surrounding the city letting nobody in or out; the churches full of groaning crowds [...]. There is nothing of that today; cholera comes to us in an age of philanthropy, unbelief, newspapers, and practical administration [...].

— CHATEAUBRIAND, *Memoirs from Beyond the Grave* (1848–50)

THE EPIDEMIC LASTED from April until November. The first victim was a dissolute sailor, carried into the Hôtel-Dieu from a ship waiting to load, down in the harbour. The man's death was public knowledge within hours. This was what everyone had been dreading, the first ambiguous sign. Cholera was already confirmed in Paris. Now it was on its way to Rouen.

In the collective imagination, fired by anxious talk, the thing was already within the walls, hovering over the city, searching for a street, looking for a suitably receptive body to take hold of. In the Hôtel-Dieu, the physicians decided to keep quiet for the moment. There had only been three cases, isolated and uncertain. The disease might yet be contained.[1]

On 10 April 1832, a steamship arrived from Paris with one hundred passengers. A sailor from the ship died of cholera, in the Hôtel-Dieu, within sixteen hours. On the same evening, there came news of multiple cases from all across the city and the suburbs. The clinical picture of cholera is memorably dramatic. It begins abruptly and runs its whole course within a week. In the first twenty-four hours there is copious but painless diarrhoea, ten litres or more. Vomiting and dehydration follow. The skin becomes cold and withered. The face is drawn and the pulse weakens. The limbs are locked as the muscles go into spasm. Death comes with a stupefied burning thirst. In 1832, the year of the epidemic, there was no effective treatment for cholera, no understanding of how it was transmitted and no coherent policy for managing the social chaos that it brought in its wake.

Cholera was a crisis of medical authority. It also provoked a political crisis. There was fear and panic below, ignorance and prejudice above, and this combination spawned rumours almost as virulent in their effects as the disease itself. Class hatred was inflamed to fantastic dimensions. The pious said that it was a punishment from God for having deposed the rightful king, Charles X, in July 1830. The destitute said it was a plot to exterminate the poor, a plot by the rich, by the government, by the doctors. They were putting poison in the bread they gave to the hungry. Provincial crowds turned against the medical students sent from Paris to help the local doctors. Any educated stranger might be part of the plot. Suspicious characters were lynched on the streets. Whole populations fled into the surrounding countryside. The National Guard was posted to protect drinking fountains and to drive away gangs of fugitives arriving from neighbouring villages. Prefects worried that the poison rumours might be the work of malevolent agitators. The editors of provincial newspapers were prosecuted for exaggerating the scale of the epidemic. Doctors disagreed bitterly with each other over the mode of the disease's transmission.

Dr Eugène Hellis, the deputy medical director of the Hôtel-Dieu, treated most of the local cases of cholera. He kept meticulous records and performed many post-mortem dissections. If anyone could understand cholera, it had to be Hellis. His book on the subject, published promptly in 1833, is entitled *Le Choléra à Rouen en 1832*. The title is deliberately prosaic. Pious Catholic though he is, Hellis refuses to exploit the fear, the horror and the grief that still lingered in the imagination of every survivor. The book is a model of evidence-based medical research, as practised in the 1830s by a physician trained in the emergent discipline of public hygiene. Working from an abundance of primary data, both narrowly clinical and broadly social, Hellis analyses the complex local patterns of mortality. The analysis, though comprehensively conceived by gender, by age, by occupation, by street, by month and by the weather, produces no firm conclusions.

There are so many anomalies, so much that remains stubbornly inexplicable. Some parts of the city, for instance, are untouched. The new houses on the harbour, the large stone houses with their cellars a good distance from the river, these have all escaped; then there is a cluster of cases along the left bank of the river, always an unhealthy part of town, with small houses near the water, subject to flooding. Cholera seems to strike at the poor and the elderly. Very few persons of quality have been affected. Many people believe, on very slender evidence, that drink is a factor. On the other hand, fear, indignation and anger appear to play a part. 'A man starts a quarrel with one of his neighbours, and cholera sets in immediately.'[2]

Perplexed by the conflicting evidence from his clinical work, Hellis refuses to believe in the contagion theory that is being advanced in certain quarters. Consequently, he opposes all isolation measures and allows cholera cases to be placed in the general medical wards. He reassures his staff that there is no point in worrying about the cholera. Either it gets you or it doesn't. If it gets you, then either you die or you don't. To their credit, the staff all stay wonderfully calm and none of them contracts the disease.[3]

Even to the least compassionate, it is obvious that the poor have it worst of all. Condemned to live in damp housing, on a poor diet and without adequate clothing, fortified by ignorance and despair, they often feel that death is no great matter. Sympathetic to their plight, Hellis asserts that he has seen the material conditions of textile workers getting rapidly worse in recent years. He dates the changes from the early 1820s. The elderly and infirm used to be cared for at home. It was a matter of working-class family pride to do so. Every year since then, competitive pressures have been driving wages down. Families fall into poverty. The offices of charitable organisations are besieged by the needy. In 1827, overwhelmed by local demand, the Hôtel-Dieu had decreed that all beds would henceforth be reserved for residents of the city alone.

Colloquially, this incomprehensible thing is *le fleau*, the scourge, a word that carries a great catastrophic payload of guilt, punishment and mortification. For all his careful statistics, Hellis acknowledges that cholera remains a mystery. 'It escapes us, it defies our calculations, our investigations; it is inscrutable; we have no purchase on it, no strategy, since we are ignorant of its nature and its laws, and we are incapable of saying for sure whether it is present or not.'[4] In this plight, magical thinking takes hold of even the educated mind, and perhaps one's statistics are only a kind of charm designed to ward off the general contagion. 'People insisted that cholera was simply uncanny, and everyone liked to dress it up as something miraculous and astonishing.'[5]

A wild abundance of remedies, both material and spiritual, were devised and debated. 'Everyone', writes Hellis, 'was a doctor, apart from the doctor himself. Some prepared baths and fumigations; others […] mixed a superlative punch; there was much making of sachets and poultices, much counting of leeches; marvellous viols containing balms and ethers, camphors and medicinal oils were arrayed artistically in little boxes.'[6] In this atmosphere, charlatans prospered, doctors squabbled and priests evoked the wrath of God. Catholic editorials denounced 'a government and a people who in the face of death only know to seek help in pharmacies'. Meanwhile secular officials organised the washing of public squares with chlorine and urged citizens to take warm baths while drinking hot tea.[7]

The long-rumbling quarrel between religion and science would rumble on for at least another generation. The inability of qualified physicians to combat the epidemic of 1832 tarnished the reputation of a supposedly omniscient profession; the gleefully punitive tone of the clergy confirmed the anti-clericalism of the secular elite. Neither side had prevailed.

Their persistent confrontation is evoked in satiric mode towards the end of *Madame Bovary* when the village pharmacist and the village priest, Homais and Bournisien, scold each other as they keep vigil over the corpse of Emma Bovary. At the height of the altercation, Homais plays his highest cards, telling the priest to

> 'Read Voltaire! … read Holbach, read the *Encyclopédie*.' […]
> They were excited, they were red-faced, they were both talking at once, heedlessly; Bournisien was shocked at such audacity; Homais was astonished at such stupidity; and they were near to trading insults […].[8]

Meanwhile, as these two rival authorities confronted one another, new and benevolent forms of social control were being refined. The epidemic of 1832 was an opportunity to implement secular bureaucratic public health policies.[9]

NOMINATED BY THE MAYOR, the marquis de Martainville, and approved by the prefect, in 1826 Achille-Cléophas was appointed to the new regional sanitary Commission. Four years later, very little had been accomplished. Critics declared that it was merely a debating club, meeting infrequently and conducting no real business. In 1831, a report was commissioned and delivered to a session of the Société libre d'émulation de Rouen, an actively philanthropic organ of the local elite. The major problem was the lack of agreement on the question of whether or not the members of the Commission should be paid. Should it be an honorary position or was there simply too much work for the original twelve nominees?

Given the size of Rouen, 'a town so populous, so large, so rich in sources of insalubriousness',[10] the report suggests that there ought to be a large number on the Commission, to spread the work. Three doctors and three chemists will need to be consulted every day, to investigate fake remedies and toxic foodstuffs. The Commission will have a remit to investigate every potential source of the insalubrious:

> the cleaning of rivers, sewers, wells, public latrines, precautions in emptying cesspools, pits, etc. […] muddy roads, slaughterhouse pits, veterinary premises, the cleaning of streets and outskirts of the city, visiting the dead, embalming, burials, cemeteries, floods, aid to the drowned, the asphyxiated and injured, fumigation chambers; markets for food and for livestock, […], slaughterhouses, […] depots for natural and artificial mineral waters, cleanliness of public and medical bath houses, nursing homes, weaning homes, houses of prostitution, public buildings, such as churches, passages, theaters, etc. […], prisons, hospitals, factories, workhouses […].[11]

The list is magnificently ambitious. The reality was disappointingly modest. Rouen's Conseil de salubrité (sanitary council), finally established in August 1831 with Achille-Cléophas as its first president, was only ever consultative. All statutory authority remained with the prefect. The problem went deep. Historian William Coleman has argued convincingly that the French public health movement of the 1830s was 'closely allied to emerging industrial interests yet uncovered social facts that prompted criticism of industrialization'.[12] Enlightenment deferred: such was the reality of the age. Achille-Cléophas was nominated for his Legion of Honour in May 1833. We may wonder if it clouded his vision. He was in his late forties and the honour probably came to him once a colleague with influence in high places made representations on his behalf to the liberal government that had come to power in the summer of 1830. Dr Jules Cloquet is the obvious suspect. He was an ex-student and a close friend, and he was comfortably installed near to metropolitan sources of patronage.

16

Last Rites

AFTER THE AWARD of the Legion of Honour in 1833, the archival record for Achille-Cléophas is increasingly meagre. His working life, though it was routinely demanding, year by year became insidiously less rewarding. From the deferential testimony of one of his colleagues, we can follow him on a daily ward round. 'Surrounded by a large cortege of students, sometimes joined by physicians from abroad, and often by physicians from the city or from the surrounding area, who came, as they put it, to drink once again from the source, thus accompanied he toured each of the wards, stopping at each bed to visit all of his patients one by one. Here he was in his element; this was where you had to see him to know the man […]'.[1]

The working day extended well into the night. From the same source, we know that 'however late it was, however tired he was, even when he had just returned from one of the long journeys that his profession so often required, he insisted on making the effort, and he would set off on his own, very quietly, to check once more all the silent wards of his hospital, where a patient, tormented by anxiety and insomnia, awaited him with the hope that his presence would relieve his suffering.'[2]

This admirably conscientious sense of clinical responsibility was equally and ambiguously a desire to retain a perfect monopoly of clinical authority. Because he didn't trust any of his subordinates, Achille-Cléophas rarely delegated and hardly ever took a holiday. This also meant that he never wrote The Book. This was a delicate issue. For many years he had been recording clinical material: 'a mass of observations that would have furnished ample substance for the construction of one of those monuments which science has the right to expect from such a man'.[3] In the event, he did not have time even to sketch out the plan of the book. It was in his mind that one day he would step down and hand over the position of chief surgeon to his older son. *Then* he would dedicate himself to the task of writing the book that he expected of himself.

In the interim, the more immediate gratifications of clinical work prevailed. His patients 'loved him little short of idolatry'. As recorded by one of his students, we can describe two such cherished moments of his being visibly adored. In the first instance, only hours after an operation, evidently still in great pain, one of his male patients is gazing longingly at Achille-Cléophas as he visits his bed. Their dialogue was memorably affecting to those who witnessed it.

- What do you want, dear fellow? A glass of wine? A bit of fresh air?
- No, I want …
- What is it?
- Oh I would so like to kiss you!

Achille-Cléophas promptly kisses the patient. Considering that the man's face is still covered in blood, he kisses him quite convincingly.

On another occasion, a woman arrives for a consultation. She pushes through the crowd of students. She is trembling and there are tears in her eyes. Her face is shining with happiness and gratitude. She cannot find the words to say it. She stammers, she falls to her knees and she takes hold of the hand that performed the operation, covering it with her tears and her kisses. 'He had cured this woman […] and she had come to pay him with the gold that she held in her heart.'[4]

The patients were not the problem. His family and his colleagues were the problem. An incident that took place around the time of the award of the Legion of Honour illustrates the difficulty of this the mature phase of his career. His older son Achille foolishly failed his medical exams in Paris. In a state of growing exasperation, Achille-Cléophas took him in hand, gave him anatomy lessons and kept a close eye on his progress. On the day that Achille so belatedly qualified, there was a small explosion of paternal rage. Gustave Flaubert said that Achille-Cléophas shook his fist at Achille and said: 'If I had been in your place, at your age, with the money you have, what a man I would have been!' The story is probably distorted. It comes from Gustave, who disliked his older brother. On the other hand, the alleged utterance seems perfectly in character. Mediocrity was intolerable to Achille-Cléophas.

The disparaging remark itself may well have been transposed. He may have said it behind his son's back, to his wife. Overheard by an envious younger son, it could then be fitted into a more overtly aggressive scenario in which the father is overwhelmed by contempt for his disappointing son and heir.[5]

The 1830s were further marked by acrimonious relations with many of his immediate colleagues. Even the best of doctors will sometimes acknowledge, in confidence, the fact that *you only have so many years of medicine in you*. From the evidence available, Achille-Cléophas appears to have reached that limit relatively early, at some point in his late forties. He is henceforth involved in various bitterly personal campaigns to defend prerogatives and interests long since acquired. In the process, Achille-Cléophas became the object of 'epigrams more or less malicious.' Things were turning sour all around him. Having now accumulated a substantial fortune, he was enviously portrayed as a money-grabber. 'Independent and somewhat obstinate', he resisted the various structural reforms that would have deprived him of some portion of his lucrative domain.

Even Dr Védie, the admiring biographer-colleague, laments the fact that Achille-Cléophas refused to step aside in time. 'He who had done everything for his hospital, he who had lavished upon it all the affection that he did not give to his family; he, the idol of his patients who loved him fanatically, whilst he was still in good health, still full of moral and intellectual energy, he ought to have passed on to others a burden evidently too heavy for him to bear [...]'.[6]

IN THE SUMMER OF 1840, at the age of fifty-five, after many years of struggling to sustain the enterprise, Achille-Cléophas resigned as the director of the medical school.[7] Several difficulties were conspiring, ominously, to confound a man hitherto so indefatigable in the pursuit of his profession.

Achille-Cléophas was locked in conflict with his formerly admiring deputy, Dr Émile Leudet. Their quarrel had been simmering ever since 1834, when the deputies in both the surgical and the medical divisions had complained of being treated unjustly by their superiors.[8] In Leudet's account of his professional relations with Achille-Cléophas, he had pursued his medical training in Rouen and had become particularly attached to Achille-Cléophas on account of his talent and his kindness. In 1820, after the resignation of his current surgical deputy, Achille-Cléophas had proposed and supported Leudet for this post, in preference to Hellis, the official nominee. Thereafter though, according to Leudet, Achille-Cléophas had refused to delegate even minor clinical responsibility, starving him of essential practical experience.

It was hinted that the chief surgeon was clinging to his prerogatives for financial reasons. Leudet declared that he could no longer continue as a deputy and offered his resignation. This was refused by the prefect. At this point, Achille-Cléophas had led Leudet to believe that some more equitable arrangement could be negotiated. Evidently, such an arrangement never emerged. We know this from an aside in one of Gustave Flaubert's letters, lamenting the fact that in the summer of 1839 the family will be confined to Rouen, because 'my father does not want that scoundrel Leudet visiting *his* patients.'[9]

On top of this quarrel, Achille-Cléophas failed to prevent a major reorganisation of the Hôtel-Dieu that deprived him of a significant portion of his clinical authority. In August 1837, the Commission proposed a reorganisation of the medical and the surgical divisions. The heads of both divisions would henceforth share responsibilities with a deputy. Both heads opposed the measure, as being to their detriment. The Commission compromised, allowing the current heads to retain their titles, their salaries and their lodgings. Even so, the reform was carried through in 1840. Achille-Cléophas responded by resigning as head of the medical school.

IN JUNE 1844 DR FLAUBERT bought a *property* (his son's mischievous emphasis) situated out at Croisset, a cluster of houses a few miles downstream from Rouen, just around the first bend in the river. Expensive, though scarcely an extravagance, it was a large handsome old property of the kind that any big man of medicine might acquire in the closing years of a triumphantly lucrative career. Croisset, his just reward, stood on the right bank of the river Seine. It had spacious terraced gardens with an avenue of lime trees (where Pascal had once walked) and an open aspect to the south-east. The low white eighteenth-century house looked out onto the great silver-grey curve of the river, little wooded islands out in the stream and the green meadows of Normandy beyond. Only half an hour away by paddle-steamer from the malodorous streets, the raw smoking chimneys and the snorting, lunging industrial engines of nineteenth-century Rouen, Croisset was the pleasant rural face of the bourgeois century.

Achille-Cléophas was not to enjoy it for very long. By November 1845, after suffering in silence for months, he was obviously too ill and too tired to work effectively. 'Premature signs of ageing had made their appearance, over the previous few years, both in his appearance and in his movements.'[10] He walked like a man bent beneath a great burden. His limbs were heavy and he staggered as if he were drunk. On Saturday 10 November 1845 he did his usual ward round at the Hôtel-Dieu. He taught his students and performed all his regular duties. That evening when he returned to Croisset he was exhausted. He had no appetite and he seemed broken in body and mind. Next day, acknowledging his condition, he had himself carried into Rouen, to the Hôtel-Dieu, and put himself into the care of his elder son.

A deep abscess was discovered in his thigh. In a rare moment of clumsiness, Achille-Cleophas must have dropped his scalpel whilst dissecting a corpse. It was the accident that every surgeon dreaded. The contaminated blade had pierced his skin, inflicting a tiny wound that had now grown into this secret horror. Drastic measures were required to save the man's life. Dr Flaubert called upon his two closest friends, Dr Cloquet and Dr Marjolin. They were fellow-surgeons, men who had studied with him. They agreed what had to be done. The only hope was to cut open the great abscess, drain the pus from the cavity in the thigh muscle and then simply trust in the body's natural powers of recovery.

But who was to perform the operation? Cloquet or Marjolin? It was impossible to decide. Who was going to concede the superiority of the other? Professional etiquette. Personal loyalty. Self-importance. There was too much at stake. Dr Flaubert resolved the issue. He decreed that his son, Achille, would hold the scalpel.

The surgeon's hand trembled for a second but then moved decisively. The blade of the knife cut deep into the leg. For some days, there was hope. Then it became clear that it was too late to save him. The news of his condition was soon made public knowledge. In the final weeks, as was proper for a high-bourgeois deathbed, the magistrate, the mayor and the archbishop, as well as colleagues, friends and ex-patients, arrived to pay their respects and to say farewell. After ten weeks, worn out by persistent vomiting, Achille-Cléophas died of septicaemia, at the age of sixty-one, on 15 January 1846, 'at half past ten in the morning, in the midst of those he had loved so much'.[11]

IN ITS DETAILED REPORT of the funeral, the *Journal de Rouen* amplified the collective emotions of the hour, turning this death into a public event of a rare solemnity. A large crowd, including all classes of the population, filled the nearby church, the Église de la Madeleine, to say a last farewell to the worthy man, the enlightened physician. The immense neo-classical church interior was draped in black, the work of a group of his former students. The coffin was carried into the church on the shoulders of a group of harbourmen. They had written to the widow, a letter both noble and moving, requesting the honour of carrying their benefactor's coffin from the mortuary into the church.

After the funeral mass, the coffin was placed on a carriage, along with the black drapes. As a member of the Legion of Honour, Achille-Cléophas was entitled to formal military honours. Accordingly, a detachment of troops of the line formed part of the cortege that made its way along the boulevards and up to the monumental cemetery. At the graveside, there were speeches, 'interrupted by the emotion of the orators, an emotion shared by all present', a unanimity of feeling that did credit to all parties. There was to be a public subscription to erect a funeral monument to his memory, to stand in the Hôtel-Dieu.

It was a curious feature of the bourgeois culture of the day that elaborate public religious funerals were common, even for Voltaireans of a decorously muted anti-clericalism. For a citizen of Achille-Cléophas's status and reputation it was the proper way. The occasion required hangings and ornaments, a funeral car with flowers, pulled by horses in fancy trappings, a cortege of family, friends and dependants crossing the city, speeches at the graveside to be printed in the newspapers, a pamphlet with portrait and biography, a public monument and perhaps a street renamed in his honour.

The building in which the funeral mass took place was the chapel for the Hôtel-Dieu. Built in the late eighteenth century in the monumental neo-classical idiom, it could easily double as a temple of reason. The frieze on the massive triangular pediment at the top of the façade features the unmistakeable Enlightenment motif of sunbeams parting the clouds.

The monumental cemetery, where Achille-Cléophas was buried, was of more recent vintage. Opened in 1828, in emulation of Père Lachaise in Paris, the cemetery offered to persons of quality an array of nice distinctions of status, along with a whole portfolio of architectural styles, Greek, Egyptian, Roman and Renaissance. Contemplating the pyramid, the obelisk, the column, the sarcophagus, even a perpetual Voltairean might find rest here, beneath an emblem both imposing and congenial.[12]

Epilogue

The last word belongs to Gustave Flaubert, the famous son of the enlightened physician. Towards the end of *Madame Bovary*, as Emma lies dying, attended by bickering medical incompetents, the famous Dr Larivière arrives on the scene. Larivière is a portrait of Achille-Cléophas.

He belonged to the great school of surgery that sprang up around Bichat, to that generation, now extinct, of philosopher-practitioners who, cherishing their art with fanatical passion, exercised it with exaltation and sagacity. Everyone in his hospital used to tremble when Larivière lost his temper, and such was his students' veneration for him that they endeavoured, as soon as they were set up in practice, to imitate him as closely as possible; thus you saw them, in the local towns, with the same long merino overcoat and loose black jacket that he always wore, with the unbuttoned cuffs half covering his plump hands, such beautiful hands, and never gloved, as though in even greater readiness to plunge into wretchedness. Disdaining medals, titles and academic honours, hospitable, generous, a father to the poor, a man who practised virtue without believing in it, he might almost have passed for a saint had not the keenness of his intellect made him feared like a demon. His gaze, slicing more cleanly than his scalpel, went right down into your soul and dissected the lies swathed in discretion and pretence. And so he went about his business, full of the majestic affability that comes of the consciousness of great talent, wealth and forty irreproachable years of hard work.[1]

Notes

PREFACE: CHILDREN OF NAPOLEON

1   J. Cloquet, *Fragments de divers memoirs*. Ms. 1055. Paris: Bibliothèque de l'Académie de Médecine, 1842, f. 21.
2   G. Flaubert, *Correspondance: Volume Three*, ed. Jean Bruneau. Paris: Gallimard, 1991, 881.

CHAPTER 1: ANCIEN RÉGIME

1   C. Jones, *The Great Nation: France from Louis XV to Napoleon*. London: Allen Lane, 2002, 425.
2   Ibid., 326.
3   C. Jones, *The Longman Companion to the French Revolution*. London: Longman, 1988, 247 & 282.
4   P. Bourdieu, 'Forms of Capital' in *Handbook for Theory and Research for the Sociology of Education*, ed. J.G. Richardson. London: Greenwood Press, 1986, 46–58.
5   K. Marx, *The Revolutions of 1848*. Harmondsworth: Penguin Books, 1973, 70.
6   A.L.J. Railliet and L. Moul, *Histoire de l'École d'Alfort*. Paris: Asselin et Houzeau, 1908, 751–6.
7   Railliet and Moul, *Histoire de l'École d'Alfort*, 541.
8   Ibid., 600.
9   J.E. Lesch, *Science and Medicine in France: The Emergence of Experimental Physiology 1790–1855*. Cambridge, MA: Harvard University Press, 1984, 28.
10 Railliet and Moul, *Histoire de l'École d'Alfort*, 49.
11 Ibid., 54.

12 G. Dubosc, *Trois Normands: Pierre Corneille, Gustave Flaubert, Guy de Maupassant; études documentaires*. Rouen: H. Defontaine, 1917, 99–101.

13 Ibid., 100.

14 Railliet and Moul, *Histoire de l'École d'Alfort*, 602.

15 F. Lebrun, 'Amour et mariage' in *Histoire de la population française*, ed. J. Dupaquier. Paris: Presses universitaires de France, 1988. Volume 2: 294–316.

16 M. Reibel, *Les Flaubert: vétérinaires champenois et l'origine de Gustave Flaubert*. Troyes: Imprimerie Gustave Fremont, 1913, 7.

17 T. Curtis, 'Nogent-sur-Seine' in *The London Encyclopaedia: or, Universal Dictionary of Science*. Volume 15. London: Thomas Tegg, 1829, 15: 69.

18 Flaubert, *Œuvres complètes*: Volume Two: 42.

19 R. Tombs, *France 1814–1914*. London: Longman, 1996, 331.

20 *Journal de l'Empire*, 2 March 1814.

21 M. Collin, *Notes historiques sur le canton de Nogent-sur-Seine: Annuaire administratif et statistique de l'Aube pour 1836*. Paris: le Livre d'histoire, 2004, 15: 691.

22 Flaubert, *Correspondance: Volume Three*, 1557.

23 Flaubert, *Correspondance: Volume One*, 68.

24 Flaubert, *Correspondance: Volume Two*, 430.

25 A. Védie, *Notice biographique sur M. Flaubert, chirurgien en chef de l'Hotel-Dieu de Rouen*. Rouen, Imprimerie de D. Briere, 1847, 5.

26 Ibid., 8.

CHAPTER 2: FRESH CORPSES

1 P. Bru, *Histoire de Bicêtre*. Paris: Lecrosnié & Babé, 1890, 87–8.

2 Ibid.

3 Reibel, *Les Flaubert*, 8.

4 Tombs, *France 1814–1914*, 10.

5 R. Finnegan, 'Family Myths, Memories and Interviewing' in *The Oral History Reader*, ed. R.T. Perks. London: Routledge, 2006.

6 Flaubert, *Correspondance: Volume One*, 347.

7 F. Clérembault, 'Le champenois Nicolas Flaubert' in *Causeries documentées, lues en des Réunions privées*. Rouen: A. Lestrignant, 1912, 20.

8 Jones, *The Longman Companion to the French Revolution*, 122.

9 Clérembault, 'Le champenois Nicolas Flaubert', 21.

10 P. McPhee, *Living the French Revolution 1789–1799*. Basingstoke: Palgrave Macmillan, 2006, 133.

11 Ibid., 148.

12 Jones, *The Great Nation*, 478.

13 *Réimpression de l'Ancien Moniteur* 19, 216.

14 Ibid., 612.

15 G. Dubosc, 'Les Ancêtres paternels de Gustave Flaubert', *Journal de Rouen* (17 février 1924).

16 H. Wallon, *Histoire du tribunal révolutionnaire de Paris*. Paris: Hachette, 1880, 2: 190.

17 Wallon, *Histoire du tribunal révolutionnaire de Paris*, 2: 250.

18 Ibid., 2: 528.

19 Clérembault, 'Le champenois Nicolas Flaubert', 23–4.

20 R. Cobb and C. Jones, *The French Revolution: Voices from a Momentous Epoch*. London: Simon and Schuster, 1988, 179.

21 Ibid., 135.

22 Dubosc, 'Les Ancêtres paternels de Gustave Flaubert'.

23 Bru, *Histoire de Bicêtre*, 101.

24 J. Legrand, *Chronicle of the French Revolution*. London: Longman, 1989, 441, 445, 453.

25 Clérembault, 'Le champenois Nicolas Flaubert', 24.

26 M.A. Petit, 'Discours sur l'influence de la Révolution française sur la santé publique' in *Essai sur la médecine du cœur*. Paris: Garnier, Reymann, 1806, 151–4.

27 P. Pinel, *A Treatise on Insanity*. London: Cadell and Davies, 1806, 68–70.

CHAPTER 3: A RADICAL EDUCATION

1 C. Commainville, *Souvenirs intimes* (1926) <http://flaubert.univ-rouen.fr/biographie/caroline/intimes.php> accessed 20 August 2011, xiv.

2 'Vue du Collège et d'une partie des murailles de Sens' (1823), courtesy of La Société archaéologique de Sens.

3 S. Desan, *Reclaiming the Sacred: Lay Religon and Popular Politics in Revolutionary France*. Ithaca, NY: Cornell University Press, 1990, 69.

4 E. Dodet, *Sens au XIXe siècle: L'essor de l'enseignement*. Sens: Société Archéologique de Sens, 2001, 49.

5 Ibid., 22.

6 Ibid., 27.

7 Ibid., 49.

8 Desan, *Reclaiming the Sacred*, 51.

9 Robertson, *France: Blue Guide*, 611.

10 Dodet, *Sens au XIXe siècle*, 26.

11 Desan, *Reclaiming the Sacred*, 55.
12 Jones, *The Longman Companion to the French Revolution*, 244.
13 Dodet, *Sens au XIXe siècle*, 26.
14 Poitevin. *Catéchisme républicain suivi de maximes de morale propre à l'éducation des enfans de l'un et de l'autre sexe*. Paris: chez Millet, 1794, 1.
15 Dodet, *Sens au XIXe siècle*, 27.
16 Ibid., 26.
17 Védie, *Notice biographique sur M. Flaubert*, 6.
18 Ibid., 6.
19 Dodet, *Sens au XIXe siècle*, 36–7.
20 Desan, *Reclaiming the Sacred*, 90.
21 *Almanac de la commune de Sens pour l'année quatrième de la République française*. Sens: Chez Veuve Tarbé & fils, 1796, 66.
22 J.B. Salgues, *Troisième mémoire pour l'infortuné Lesurques*. Paris: Imprimerie de Auguste Mie, 1829, 176.
23 Ibid., 177.
24 Ibid., 177–82.
25 Dodet, *Sens au XIXe siècle*, 38.

CHAPTER 4: READING VOLTAIRE

1 F.N. Benoist-Lamothe, *Prospectus concernant la réouverture d'une école Senonaise*. Société Archéologique de Sens, 2007.
2 J.P. Fontaine, *Les Mysteres de l'Yonne*. Romagnat: Editions de Borée, 2005, 370.
3 Benoist de Lamothe, *Observateur* no. 8, 5 germinal an IV / 25 March 1796; cited in Mathiez, *La Théophilanthropie et le culte décadaire*, 65.
4 Ibid.
5 Ibid., 359–72.
6 Benoist-Lamothe, *Prospectus concernant la réouverture d'une école Senonaise*.
7 Voltaire, *Philosophical Dictionary*. New York: Basic Books, 1962, 56.
8 Gay, *The Party of Humanity: Studies in the French Enlightenment*, 11 & 14–15.
9 Védie, *Notice biographique sur M. Flaubert*, 23.
10 Ibid., 23.
11 R. Williams, *Marxism and Literature*. Oxford: Oxford University Press, 1977, 132.

12 D. Fauvel, *La Bibliothèque d'Achille-Cléophas Flaubert: inventaire après décès*. Rouen: Archives départmentates de la Seine-Maritime, 2005, cote 2E/8/237, recto.

13 S. Bird, *Reinventing Voltaire: The Politics of Commemoration in Nineteenth-Century France*. Oxford: Voltaire Foundation, 2000, 6.

14 Védie, *Notice biographique sur M. Flaubert*, 6–8.

15 S. Hazareesingh, *The Legend of Napoleon*. London: Granta, 2004, 106.

CHAPTER 5: PARISIANS

1 Reibel, *Les Flaubert*, 35.

2 Commainville, *Souvenirs intimes*, 3.

3 *Morning Chronicle* (London), 27 July 1802.

4 Fauvel, *La Bibliothèque d'Achille-Cléophas Flaubert*, cote 2E/8/237, acte 1590.

5 Védie, *Notice biographique sur M. Flaubert*, 7.

6 J.G. Alger, 'British Visitors to Paris, 1802–1803'. *The English Historical Review* 14.56 (1899): 739–41, 739.

7 *Morning Chronicle* (London), 14 September 1802.

8 *Morning Chronicle* (London), 28 July 1802.

9 S.L. Mitchell, *The American Repository and Review of American Publications on Medicine, Surgery, and the Auxiliary Branches of Philosophy*. New York: Faculty of Physic of Columbia College, 1802, 180.

10 W. Benjamin, *The Arcades Project*, trans. Howard Eiland and Kevin McLaughlin, ed. Rolf Tiedemann. Cambridge, MA: Belknap Press, 1999, 32.

11 Ibid., 42, 55, 56.

12 A. Fourcroy, 'Première adresse des officiers du Jardin des plantes & du Cabinet d'histoire naturelle, lue à l'Assemblée nationale, le 20 Août 1790' (1790). *The French Revolution Research Collection* <http://gallica.bnf.fr/ark:/12148/bpt6k420666/f3.image> accessed 3 October 2012, 2.

13 Ibid., 3.

14 Smellie, 'Preface by the Translator', in *Natural History General and Particular by the Count de Buffon*. London: Strahan & Cadell, 1785, I: xv–xvi.

15 Védie, *Notice biographique sur M. Flaubert*, 8.

16 *Morning Post and Gazetteer* (London), 25 September 1802.

17 Ibid.

18 *Morning Chronicle* (London), 6 August 1802.

19 *Morning Chronicle* (London), 1 November 1802.

CHAPTER 6: THE NEW SCIENCE OF MAN

1 Védie, *Notice biographique sur M. Flaubert*, 8.
2 M.S. Staum, *Cabanis: Enlightenment and Medical Philosophy in the French Revolution*. Princeton: Princeton University Press, 1980, 17–18.
3 Weiner 1969, 670.
4 Staum, *Cabanis*, 383.
5 P.J.G. Cabanis, *Coup d'œil sur les révolutions et sur la reforme de la médecine*. Paris: Crapelet, 1804, 437–8.
6 P.J.G. Cabanis, *Rapport fait au nom de la Commission d'instruction publique, et projet de résolution, sur un mode provisoire de police médicale*. Paris: C. d. Cinq-Cents, 1798, 11.
7 Cabanis, *Rapports du physique et du moral de l'homme*. Paris: Crapelet, 1805, 1: vii.
8 Ibid., 1: xl.
9 Ibid., 1: 154.
10 Cloquet, *Etudes de physiologie*. Paris: Bibliothèque de L'Académie nationale de médecine, cote 130 (1061).
11 Cabanis, *Rapports du physique et du moral de l'homme*, 1: 217.
12 Flaubert, *Correspondance: Volume One*, 326.
13 R. Maulitz, *Morbid Appearances: The Anatomy of Pathology in the Early Nineteenth Century*. Cambridge: Cambridge University Press, 1987, 1–2.
14 D. Outram, *Georges Cuvier: Vocation, Science and Authority in Post-Revolutionary France*. Basingstoke: Palgrave Macmillan, 1984, 47.
15 Petit, 'Discours sur l'influence de la Révolution française sur la santé publique', 136.
16 J.V. Pickstone, 'Bureaucracy, Liberalism and the Body in Post-Revolutionary France: Bichat's Physiology and the Paris School of Medicine', *History of Science* xix (1981): 115–42, 135.
17 D.M. Vess, *Medical Revolution in France 1789–1796*. Gainesville: University Press of Florida, 1975, 88.
18 Ibid., 74.
19 Bichat, 'Discours préliminaire', *Mémoires de la Société médicale d'émulation*. Paris: Chez Maradan, 1798, ix.

CHAPTER 7: ANATOMY LESSONS

1 M. Ramsey, *Professional and Popular Medicine in France, 1770–1830: The Social World of Medical Practice.* Cambridge: Cambridge University Press, 1988, 109.

2 E.H. Ackerknecht, *Medicine at the Paris Hospital, 1794–1848.* Baltimore: Johns Hopkins University Press, 1967, 36.

3 Védie, *Notice biographique sur M. Flaubert*, 7.

4 J.E. Lesch, *Science and Medicine in France: The Emergence of Experimental Physiology 1790–1855.* Cambridge, MA: Harvard University Press, 1984, 53.

5 Vess, *Medical Revolution in France 1789–1796*, 40.

6 Védie, *Notice biographique sur M. Flaubert*, 8.

7 Flaubert, *Correspondance: Volume Three*, 1023.

8 A. Desmond & J. Moore, *Darwin.* London: Penguin, 1992, 26–7.

9 D. Diderot and J. D'Alembert (eds), *Encyclopédie, ou dictionnaire raisonné des sciences, des arts et des métiers.* Paris: chez Briasson, 1751, 1: 409–10.

10 Ibid., 1: 410.

11 D. Parent-Duchâtelet and D'Arcet, 'De l'influence et de l'assainissement des salles de dissection', *Annales d'hygiène publique et de médecine légale* 5 (1831): 260.

12 A. Cunningham, *The Anatomist Anatomis'd: An Experimental Discipline in Enlightenment Europe.* Farnham: Ashgate, 2010, 384.

13 Vigné, 'Eloge de Laumonier', *Précis analytique des travaux de l'Académie des Sciences de Rouen.* Rouen: Periaux, 1819, 117.

14 Staum, *Cabanis*, 381.

15 J.J. Leroux, *Discours prononcé sur la tombe de M. Hallé.* Paris: Imprimerie Didot le jeune, 1822, 8.

16 G. Cuvier, *Receuil des éloges historiques.* Strasbourg: F.G. Lavraut, 1827, 3: ccx.

17 Hallé, cited in M.S. Staum, 'The Class of Moral and Political Sciences, 1795–1803', *French Historical Studies* 11.3 (1980), 381.

18 H. Klencke, *Lives of the Brothers Humboldt, Alexander and William.* New York: Harper and Brothers, 1854, 90.

19 See <www.sciencephoto.com/media/129311/view> accessed 1 October 2013.

20. A.C. Flaubert, 'Discours de réception', pages 26–9 in *Précis analytique des travaux de l'Académie Royale des sciences, des belles-lettres et des art de Rouen pendant l'année 1815.* Rouen: P. Periaux, 1815, 27–8.

21 Védie, *Notice biographique sur M. Flaubert*, 6–7.

22 G. Flaubert, *Madame Bovary*, trans. Geoffrey Wall. London: Penguin Books, 1992, 56; translation modified.

23 Flaubert, *Correspondance: Volume Two*, 295.
24 R.T. Murdoch, 'Newton and the French Muse', *Journal of the History of Ideas* 19.3, 327.

CHAPTER 8: CONSCRIPTION

1 A. Forrest, 'Conscription and Crime in Rural France during the Directory and Consulate' in *Beyond the Terror: Essays in French Regional and Social History, 1794–1815*, ed. G. Lewis and C. Lucas. Cambridge: Cambridge University Press, 1983, 116.
2 G. Daly, *Inside Napoleonic France: State and Society in Rouen, 1800–1815*. Aldershot: Ashgate, 2001, 237–42.
3 P. Berteau, 'Docteur Achille-Cléophas, chirurgien rouennais', *Bulletin Flaubert–Maupassant* 15 (2004): 13–40, 16–17.
4 W.B. Weiner, 'French Doctors Face War: 1792–1815' in *From the Ancien Régime to the Popular Front: Essays in the History of Modern France*, ed. C.K. Warner. New York: Columbia University Press, 1969: 51–73, 67–71.
5 D. Outram, *Georges Cuvier: Vocation, Science and Authority in Post-Revolutionary France*. Basingstoke: Palgrave Macmillan, 1984, 47.
6 A. Dubuc, 'La nomination du père de Flaubert, en 1806, à Hôtel-Dieu de Rouen', *Les Amis de Flaubert* 24 (1964): 43–6, 44.
7 There is substantial testimony concerning the domineering side of Dupuytren; it is my hypothesis that these published opinions are the residue of professional gossip.
8 P. Wylock, 'The Life and Times of Guillaume Dupuytren', *Canadian Journal of Surgery* 32.6 (1989): 4, 473–7.
9 Védie, *Notice biographique sur M. Flaubert*, 9.

CHAPTER 9: A CENTURY OF MARVELS

1 *Journal de Rouen*, 4 December 1806.
2 *Journal de Rouen*, 10 November 1806.
3 *Journal de Rouen*, 2 November 1806.
4 *Journal de Rouen*, 14 November 1806.
5 *Journal de Rouen*, 28 November 1806.
6 *Journal de Rouen*, 11 November 1806.
7 *Journal de Rouen*, 14 November 1806.
8 Ibid.

9   S. Chassagne, *Le Coton et ses patrons: France 1760–1840*. Paris: Éditions de l'École des Hautes Études en Sciences Sociales, 1991, 230.

10   J.P. Chaline, *Les Bourgeois de Rouen: une élite urbaine au XIXe siècle*. Paris: Presse de la Fondation Nationale des Sciences Politiques, 1982, 119–20; J.P. Chaline, 'The Cotton Manufacturer in Normandy and England During the Nineteenth Century'. *Textile History* 17.1 (1986): 19–25.

11   Chaline, *Les Bourgeois de Rouen*, 261.

12   D.M.P. Hellis, *Clinique médicale de l'Hôtel-Dieu de Rouen*. Paris: Chez Gabon, 1826, 41–2.

13   J. Marchand, 'L'apothicairerie de l'Hôtel Dieu de Rouen et ses apothicaires', Groupe Histoire des Hôpitaux de Rouen, Journées du Patrimoine du 14 septembre 2006 <http://www3.chu-rouen.fr/NR/rdonlyres/B1DAD9ED-C86D-4B07-A58C-5AC957015388/0/2006_marchand.pdf> accessed 3 October 2012, 1–7.

14   Daly, *Inside Napoleonic France*, 29.

15   A. Floquet, 'Bordier & Jourdain', *Histoire du Parlement de Normandie: Vol VII*. Rouen: Édouard frères, 1842: 554–65, 7: 555.

16   Pennetier, *Le Chirurgien Laumonier*. Rouen: Imprimerie Julien Lecerf, 1887, 28.

17   *Journal de Rouen* (14 January 1818).

CHAPTER 10: COMPASSIONATE KNOWLEDGE

1   Pennetier, *Le Chirurgien Laumonier*, 8.

2   Védie, *Notice biographique sur M. Flaubert*, 10.

3   Cloquet, *Études de physiologie*, 1.

4   Ibid., 3.

5   Ibid., 4.

6   Ibid., 8.

7   Ibid., 9.

8   Ibid., 9.

9   Ibid., 11.

10   Ibid., 10.

11   Ibid., 12.

12   Ibid., 11.

13   Ibid., 16.

14   Ibid., 18–19.

15   Ibid., 27.

16   Ibid., 28.

17 Flaubert 1810, v.
18 Flaubert, *Correspondance: Volume Two*, 292.
19 Pennetier, *Le Chirurgien Laumonier*, 14.
20 Védie, *Notice biographique sur M. Flaubert*, 11.
21 A.-C. Flaubert, *Dissertation sur la manière de conduire les malades avant et après les opérations chirurgicales*. Paris: Didot Jeune, 1810, 16.
22 Ibid., 27.
23 Ibid., 46.
24 Ibid., 50.
25 Ibid., 22.
26 Ibid., 47.
27 Ibid., 18.
28 Ibid., 15.
29 Ibid., 65.
30 A. Dubois, 'Achille-Cléophas Flaubert', *Bulletin Flaubert–Maupassant* 15 (2004): 40–7, 44.

CHAPTER 11: HEIRESS AND ORPHAN

1 D. Fauvel, 'Achille-Cléophas Flaubert d'après les registres de l'Hôtel Dieu', *Bulletin Flaubert–Maupassant* 15 (2004): 61.
2 F. Brown, *Flaubert: A Life*. Cambridge, MA: Harvard University Press, 2007, 19.
3 Commainville, *Souvenirs intimes*.
4 Ibid.
5 Chaline, *Les Bourgeois de Rouen*, 110.
6 Chaline, *Les Bourgeois de Rouen*, 214.
7 Flaubert, *Correspondance: Volume One*, 369.
8 Ibid., 86, 129, 151, 170, 198, 216.
9 Flaubert, *Correspondance: Volume Two*, 100.
10 B.F. Bart, *Flaubert*. Syracuse, NY: Syracuse University Press, 1967, 178.

CHAPTER 12: LOYALTIES

1 E. Badinter and R. Badinter, *Condorcet: un intellectuel en politique*. Paris: Fayard, 1988; C. Gillespie, *Science and Polity in France: The Revolutionary and Napoleonic Years*. Princeton: Princeton University Press, 2004, 330–11.

2   Condorcet, 'Sketch for a Historical Picture of the Progress of the Human Mind: Tenth Epoch', trans. Keith Baker. *Daedalus* 133.3 (1795): 65–82, 64.

3   Ibid., 69.

4   L. Chevalier, *Classes laborieuses et classes dangereuses*. Paris: Plon, 1958.

5   B.M. Ratcliffe, 'Classes laborieuses et classes dangereuses à Paris: The Chevalier Thesis Reexamined', *French Historical Studies* 17.2 (1991): 542–74.

6   Y. Marec, *Pauvreté et protection sociale aux XIXe et XXe siècles*. Rennes: Presses universitaires de Rennes, 2006.

7   D. Fauvel, 'Achille-Cléophas d'après les registres de l'Hôtel-Dieu', *Bulletin Flaubert–Maupassant* 15 (2004): 59–70, 59.

8   Ibid., 62.

9   A.-C. Flaubert, letter dated 28 June 1815. Photocopy, courtesy of Yvan Leclerc.

10   Fauvel, 'Achille-Cléophas d'après les registres de l'Hôtel-Dieu', 62.

11   L. Andrieu, 'La Nomination du père de Flaubert comme Chirurgien-Chef'. *Les Amis de Flaubert* 37 (1967): 38–42, 38.

12   Ibid., 39.

13   Tombs, *France 1814–1914*, 10.

14   Andrieu, 'La Nomination du père de Flaubert comme Chirurgien-Chef', 39–40.

15   Fauvel, 'Achille-Cléophas d'après les registres de l'Hôtel-Dieu', 64.

16   *Journal de Rouen*, 14–17 June 1825.

17   Flaubert, *Correspondance: Volume One*, 76.

CHAPTER 13: FUTURE PERFECT

1   C.E. Harrison, *The Bourgeois Citizen in Nineteenth-Century France*. Oxford: Oxford University Press, 1999, 64–5.

2   *Précis analytique des travaux de l'Académie Royale des sciences, des belles-lettres et des arts de Rouen pendant l'année 1825*. Rouen: P. Periaux, 1825, 215.

3   Académie 1827, 180–3.

4   Académie 1818, 27.

5   Académie 1816, XXX.

6   A. Thiers, *Histoire de la Révolution française. Huitième édition*. Brussels: Adolphe Wahlen, 1836, 255.

7   Tombs, *France 1814–1914*, 337.

8   *Journal de Rouen*, 20 January 1831.

9   S. Kroen, 'Revolutionizing Religious Politics During the Restoration', *French Historical Studies* 21.1 (1998): 27–53, 32.

10 Ibid., 33.

11 Hazareesingh, *The Legend of Napoleon*, 57–63.

12 *Journal de Rouen*, 20 January 1822.

13 Kroen, 'Revolutionizing Religious Politics During the Restoration'.

14 Marec, *Pauvreté et protection sociale aux XIXe et XXe siècles*, 40–50.

15 J.P. Chaline, *Les Bourgeois de Rouen: Une élite urbaine au XIXe siècle*. Paris: Presse de la Fondation Nationale des Sciences Politiques, 1982, 293.

16 Marec, *Pauvreté et protection sociale aux XIXe et XXe siècles*, 58.

17 W. Coleman, *Death is a Social Disease: Public Health and Political Economy in Early Industrial France*. Madison: University of Wisconsin Press, 1982, xxv–xviii.

18 Ibid., 60.

19 M. Villermé, *Tableau de l'état physique et moral des ouvriers employés dans la manufacture de coton de laine et de soie*. Paris: Jules Renouard et cie, 1840, 148–9.

20 Marec, *Pauvreté et protection sociale aux XIXe et XXe siècles*, 25–6.

21 Ibid.

22 A.C. Flaubert, 'Achille-Cléophas Flaubert to the Members of the Administrative Commission of the Rouen Hospices' (10 November 1819). Photocopy of letter, courtesy of Yvan Leclerc.

CHAPTER 14: TWO NATIONS

1   A. Dubuc, 'L'enterrement du père de Gustave Flaubert', *Les Amis de Flaubert* 37 (1970): 34–6, 34.

2   Flaubert, *Correspondance: Volume Four*, 211.

3   H. Lottman, *Flaubert: A Biography*. London: Methuen, 1989, 13.

4   P. Berteau, *Docteurs Flaubert: père et fils*. Rouen: Éditions Bertout, 2006, 26.

5   Flaubert, *Correspondance: Volume One*, 406.

6   Flaubert, *Correspondance: Volume Four*, 1019.

7   Dubosc, *Trois Normands*, 141.

8   A.-C. Flaubert et al., *Réponse des chefs de service de santé des hôpitaux de Rouen à un mémoire publie par MM. leurs adjoints*. Rouen: impr. de E. Periaux fils aîné, 1834, 5–6.

9   Villermé, *Tableau de l'état physique et moral des ouvriers*.

10 A.C. Flaubert, 'Journal de Clinique' (1818), ten manuscript notebooks. Musée Flaubert et d'histoire de la médecine, Rouen, 6: 111.

11 Ibid., 2: 120–1.

12 Ibid., 3: 14.

13 Ibid., 4: 18.

14 Ibid., 9: 69–70.

15 Ibid., 2: 101–2.

16 Ibid., 3: 112–13.

17 Ibid., 5: 107.

18 Ibid., 10: 29.

19 H. Barbet, 'Suppression de la mendicité à Rouen', *Annuaire des cinq départements de l'ancienne Normandie publié par l' Association normand* (1841).

20 Flaubert, *Madame Bovary*, 216–17.

21 Ibid., 244.

22 Ibid., 281.

23 Ibid., 286.

24 Hellis, *Clinique médicale de l'Hôtel-Dieu de Rouen*, 17.

25 J. Hossard, 'Le Dr Hellis: médecin de l'Hôtel-Dieu de Rouen' (1998), *Groupe d'Histoire des Hôpitaux de Rouen* <http://www3.chu-rouen.fr/ NR/rdonlyres/80CEF43D-98C1-46C5-AFEF-FF4FFED5C708/0/1998.pdf> accessed 3 October 2012, 3.

26 Noiret 1836, 43–5.

27 J.N. Hallé, 'Hygiène moderne' in *Dictionnaire des sciences médicales*. U. S. d. M. e. d. Chirurgiens. Paris, Panckoucke. 22 HUM – HYG: 532–608. Paris: Panckoucke, 1818, 22: 550.

28 Flaubert, *Madame Bovary*, 24.

CHAPTER 15: FEAR AND TREMBLING

1 Hellis, *Clinique médicale de l'Hôtel-Dieu de Rouen*, 8–15.

2 Ibid., 14.

3 Ibid., 44–6.

4 Ibid., 25.

5 Ibid., 19.

6 Ibid., 72.

7 C.J. Kudlick, 'Giving is Deceiving: Cholera, Charity, and the Quest for Authority in 1832', *French Historical Studies* 18.2 (1993): 457–81, 465 & 467.

8 Flaubert, *Madame Bovary*, 270.

9 Kudlick, 'Giving is Deceiving', 476.

10   D.M.P. Avenel, 'Deuxième rapport sur l'établissement d'un Conseil de salubrité publique â Rouen et dans le Département de la Seine-Inférieure' in *La Société libre d'émulation de Rouen* (1830), 177.

11   Ibid., 178.

12. W. Coleman, *Death is a Social Disease: Public Health and Political Economy in Early Industrial France*. Madison: University of Wisconsin Press, 1982, 61.

CHAPTER 16: LAST RITES

1   Védie, *Notice biographique sur M. Flaubert*, 13, 18.

2   Ibid., 18.

3   Ibid., 19.

4   Ibid., 24.

5   E. Goncourt and J. Goncourt, *Pages from the Goncourt Journal*, ed. Robert Baldick. Oxford: Oxford University Press, 1962, 205.

6   Védie, *Notice biographique sur M. Flaubert*, 26–7.

7   Berteau, 'Docteur Achille-Cléophas, chirurgien rouennais', 27.

8   Flaubert, *Correspondance: Volume One*, 970; *Volume Five*, 1477.

9   Flaubert, *Correspondance: Volume One*, 46.

10   Dubuc, 'L'enterrement du père de Gustave Flaubert', 35.

11   Védie, *Notice biographique sur M. Flaubert*, 29.

12   Chaline, *Les Bourgeois de Rouen*, 287–9.

EPILOGUE

1   Flaubert, *Madame Bovary*, 262.

Bibliography

Académie de Rouen. *Précis analytique des travaux de l'Académie Royale de Rouen pendant l'année de 1816* (1817).

——. *Précis analytique des travaux de l'Académie Royale de Rouen pendant l'année de 1817* (1818).

——. *Précis analytique des travaux de l'Académie Royale de Rouen pendant l'année de 1826* (1827).

Ackerknecht, E.H. *Medicine at the Paris Hospital, 1794–1848*. Baltimore: Johns Hopkins University Press, 1967.

Ackerman, M.J. et al. *Human Anatomy: Depicting the Body from the Renaissance to Today*. London: Thames & Hudson, 2006.

Acte 1812. 20/01/1812. Délibération du Conseil de famille Fleuriot en vue mariage avec Achille Cléophas Flaubert 2E6/218.

Almanac de Sens. *Almanac de la commune de Sens pour l'année quatrième de la République française*. Sens: Chez Veuve Tarbé & fils, 1796.

Aisenberg, A.R. 'Book Review: Constructing Paris Medicine'. *Social History of Medicine* 141 (2001): 145–6.

Alger, J.G. 'British Visitors to Paris, 1802–1803'. *The English Historical Review* 14.56 (1899): 739–41.

Allard, S. *Paris 1820: L'affirmation de la génération romantique*. Oxford: Peter Lang, 2004.

Andrieu, L. 'La Nomination du père de Flaubert comme Chirurgien-Chef'. *Les Amis de Flaubert* 37 (1967): 38–42.

Armstrong, D. *A New History of Identity: A Sociology of Medical Knowledge*. London: Palgrave, 2002.

Aufauvre, A. *Histoire de Nogent-sur-Seine*. Troyes: Bouquot, 1859.

Avenel, D.M.P. 'Deuxième rapport sur l'établissement d'un Conseil de salubrité publique à Rouen et dans le Département de la Seine-Inférieure' in *La Société libre d'émulation de Rouen* (1830).

Baczko, B. *Ending the Terror: The French Revolution After Robespierre*. Cambridge: Cambridge University Press, 1994.

Badinter, E., and R. Badinter. *Condorcet: un intellectuel en politique*. Paris: Fayard, 1988.

Bailin, M. *The Sickroom in Victorian Fiction: The Art of Being Ill*. Cambridge: Cambridge University Press, 2005.

Baker, K. 'Scientism at the End of the Old Regime', *Minerva* 25 (1987): 21–34.

Barbet, H. 'Suppression de la mendicité à Rouen', *Annuaire des cinq départements de l'ancienne Normandie publié par l' Association normand* (1841).

Barry, J., and C. Jones. *Medicine and Charity Before the Welfare State*. London: Routledge, 1991.

Bashford, A., and C. Hooker. *Contagion: Historical and Cultural Studies*. London: Routledge, 2001.

Bazin, A. 'Le Choléra-Morbus à Paris' in *Paris, ou le Livre des cent et un*. Frankfurt: Schmerber, 1832: vol. 5, 209–21.

Benjamin, W. *The Arcades Project*, trans. Howard Eiland and Kevin McLaughlin, ed. Rolf Tiedemann. Cambridge, MA: Belknap Press, 1999.

Benoist-Lamothe, F.N. *Prospectus concernant la réouverture d'une école Senonaise*. Société Archéologique de Sens, 2007.

Berc, Y.M. *Le chaudron et la lancette: Croyances populaires et médicine preventive 1789–1830*. Paris: Presses de la Renaissance, 1984.

Bernis, F. de P. de. *Lettre pastorale de l'archevêque de Rouen*. Rouen: Mégard, 1819.

Berteau, P. 'Docteur Achille-Cléophas, chirurgien rouennais', *Bulletin Flaubert–Maupassant* 15 (2004): 13–40.

——. *Docteurs Flaubert: père et fils*. Rouen: Éditions Bertout, 2006.

Besterman, T. *Voltaire Essays*. Oxford: Oxford University Press, 1962.

Bezucha, R.J. *The Lyon Uprising of 1834: Social and Political Conflict in the Early July Monarchy*. Cambridge, MA: Harvard University Press, 1974.

Bichat, M.F.X. 'Discours préliminaire' in *Mémoires de la Société médicale d'émulation: 1e année: articles divers*. Paris: Chez Maradan, 1798, 1–12.

——. 'Essai sur Desault' in *Desault: Œuvres chirurgicales. Première partie: maladies des parties dures*. Paris: Vve Desault, Méquignon, Devilliers, Deroi, 1798.

——. *Recherches physiologiques sur la vie et la mort*. Paris: Brosson, Gabon, 1800.

Bird, S. *Reinventing Voltaire: The Politics of Commemoration in Nineteenth-Century France*. Oxford: Voltaire Foundation, 2000.

Blaydon, F. *Paris As It Was and As It Is*. London: C. & R. Baldwin, 1803.

Blécourt, W. de, and C. Usborne. *Cultural Approaches to the History of Medicine: Mediating Medicine in Early Modern and Modern Europe*. Basingstoke: Palgrave Macmillan, 2004.

Boisseau, F.G. 'Notice sur la vie et les travaux de Xavier Bichat' in *Anatomie pathologique, dernier cours de Xavier Bichat*. Paris: J.B. Baillière, 1825.

Bourdieu, P. 'Forms of Capital' in *Handbook for Theory and Research for the Sociology of Education*, ed. J.G. Richardson. London: Greenwood Press, 1986.

Bowler, P.J. *Evolution: The History of an Idea*. Berkeley: University of California Press, 2009.

Brockliss, L., and C. Jones. *The Medical World of Early Modern France*. Oxford: Oxford University Press, 1997.

Brown, F. *Flaubert: A Life*. Cambridge, MA: Harvard University Press, 2007.

Bru, P. *Histoire de Bicêtre*. Paris: Lecrosnié & Babé, 1890.

Buffon, G.L.L. *Natural History General and Particular*. London: A. Strahan, 1791.

Bunton, R., and A. Petersen. *Foucault, Health and Medicine*. London: Routledge, 1997.

Burkhardt, R.W. 'Lamarck, Evolution, and the Politics of Science', *Journal of the History of Biology* 3.2 (1970): 275–98.

Bynum, W.F. 'Review [untitled]', *The British Journal for the History of Science* 21.3 (1988): 369–70.

——, S. Lock et al. *Medical Journals and Medical Knowledge: Historical Essays*. London: Routledge, 1992.

Cabanes, J.L. *Le Corps et la Maladie dans les récits réalistes 1856–1893*. Paris: Klincksieck, 1991.

Cabanis, P.J.G. *Rapport fait au nom de la Commission d'instruction publique, et projet de résolution, sur un mode provisoire de police médicale*. Paris: C. d. Cinq-Cents, 1798.

——. *Coup d'œil sur les révolutions et sur la reforme de la médecine*. Paris: Crapelet, 1804.

——. *Œuvres philosophiques de Cabanis*. Paris: Presses universitaires de France, 1956.

——. *Note sur le supplice de la guillotine*. Périgueux: Fanlac, 2002.

Carette, E. *Thouret: sa vie, ses œuvres*. Paris: Picard, 1890.

Carter, E.C. *Enterprise and Entrepreneurs in Nineteenth and Twentieth-Century France*. Baltimore: Johns Hopkins University Press, 1976.

Cazort, M., M. Kornell et al. *The Ingenious Machine of Nature: Four Centuries of Art and Anatomy*. Ottawa: National Gallery of Canada, 1996.

Chaline, J.P. 'A la recherche de la bourgeoisie rouennaise du XIXe siècle', *Les Amis de Flaubert* (décembre 1969): 18–30.

——. 'Les adeptes de la théophilanthropie', *Rives nord-méditerranéennes* (put online 28 November 2005) <http://rives.revues.org/document410.html> accessed 7 July 2008.

——. *Les Bourgeois de Rouen: Une élite urbaine au XIXe siècle*. Paris: Presse de la Fondation Nationale des Sciences Politiques, 1982.

——. 'The Cotton Manufacturer in Normandy and England During the Nineteenth Century'. *Textile History* 17.I (1986): 19–26.

——. *Deux bourgeois en leur temps: documents sur la société rouennaise au XIXe siècle: textes*. Rouen, 1977.

——. 'Les rites de sociabilité chez les élites urbaines en France au XIXe siècle', *Memoria y Civilización* 3 (2000): 187–205.

——. *Sociabilité et érudition: les sociétés savantes en France: XIXe–XXe siècle*. Paris: CTHS, 1995.

——. 'Transformations urbaines et mutations économiques' in *Histoire de Rouen*, ed. M. Mollat. Toulouse: Privat, 1979.

Chaptal, A.C. *Mes souvenirs sur Napoleon*. Paris: E. Plon, Nourrit et Cie, 1893.

Chassagne, S. *Le Coton et ses patrons: France 1760–1840*. Paris: Éditions de l'École des Hautes Études en Sciences Sociales, 1991.

Choulant, L. *History and Bibliography of Anatomic Illustrations*. New York: Hafner Publishing Co., 1962.

Clérembault, F. 'Le champenois Nicolas Flaubert' in *Causeries documentées, lues en des Réunions privées*. Rouen: A. Lestrignant, 1912.

Clifford, J. *Writing Culture: The Poetics and Politics of Ethnography*. London: University of California Press, 1986.

Cloquet, G. 'Jules Cloquet: Sa vie, ses ouvres, 1790–1883', thèse de médecine no. 307. Paris: Bibliothèque nationale, 1909.

Cloquet, J. *Discours prononcé à la séance publique de la Faculté de médecine de Paris, du 3 novembre 1840*. Paris: Bignoux, 1840.

——. *Fragments de divers memoirs*. Ms. 1055. Paris: Bibliothèque de l'Académie de Médecine, 1842.

Cobb, R. *Paris and its Provinces, 1792–1802*. Oxford: Oxford University Press, 1975.

——. *The People's Armies*. New Haven and London: Yale University Press, 1987.

——. *The French and their Revolution*, ed. D. Gilmour. London: The New Press, 1999.

—— and C. Jones. *The French Revolution: Voices from a Momentous Epoch*. London: Simon and Schuster, 1988.

Coleman, W. *Death is a Social Disease: Public Health and Political Economy in Early Industrial France*. Madison: University of Wisconsin Press, 1982.

Collin, M. *Notes historiques sur le canton de Nogent-sur-Seine: Annuaire administratif et statistique de l'Aube pour 1836*. Paris: le Livre d'histoire, 2004.

Commainville, C. *Souvenirs intimes* (1926). <http://flaubert.univ-rouen.fr/ biographie/caroline/intimes.php> accessed 20 August 2011.

Condorcet. 'Sketch for a Historical Picture of the Progress of the Human Mind: Tenth Epoch', trans. Keith Baker. *Daedalus* 133.3 (1795): 65–82.

Corbin, A. *The Foul and the Fragrant: Odour and the French Social Imagination*, trans. Miriam Kochan. Cambridge, MA: Harvard University Press, 1986.

Crosland, M. *The Society of Arcueil: A View of French Science at the Time of Napoleon I*. Cambridge, MA: Harvard University Press, 1967.

——. 'The Officiers de Santé of the French Revolution: A Case Study in the Changing Language of Medicine', *Medical History* 482 (2004): 229–44.

Cross, J. *Sketches of the Medical Schools of Paris*. London: J. Callow, 1815.

Cruickshank, A.H., and E. Gaskell. 'Jean-Nicolas Marjolin: Destined to be Forgotten?'. *Medical History* 74 (1963): 383–4.

Cunningham, A. *The Anatomist Anatomis'd: An Experimental Discipline in Enlightenment Europe*. Farnham: Ashgate, 2010.

—— and B. Andrews. *Western Medicine as Contested Knowledge*. Manchester: Manchester University Press, 1997.

—— and R.K. French. *The Medical Enlightenment of the Eighteenth Century*. Cambridge: Cambridge University Press, 1990.

Curtis, T. 'Nogent-sur-Seine' in *The London Encyclopaedia: or, Universal Dictionary of Science*. Volume 15. London: Thomas Tegg, 1829.

Cuvier, G. *Rapport historique sur les progrès des sciences naturelles depuis 1789, et sur leur état actuel*. 1810.

——. *Receuil des éloges historique lues dans les séances publiques de l'Institut royal de France par M. le B. Cuvier*. Volume 3. Strasbourg: F.G. Lavraut, n.d.

Dalembert. 'Discours préliminaire des éditeurs' in *Encyclopédie Dictionnaire raisonné des Sciences, des Arts & des Métiers*. 1751.

Daly, G. *Inside Napoleonic France: State and Society in Rouen, 1800–1815*. Aldershot: Ashgate, 2001.

Darnton, R. *Mesmerism and the End of the Enlightenment in France*. Cambridge, MA: Harvard University Press, 1968.

Darnton, R. *The Business of Enlightenment: A Publishing History of the Encyclopedie 1775–1800*. Cambridge, MA: Belknap Press, 1979.

Davidson, I. *Voltaire: A Life*. London: Profile, 2010.

De Goncourt, E., and J. De Goncourt. *Histoire de la société française pendant la Révolution*. Paris: Maison Quantin, 1889.

Desmond, A., & Moore, J. *Darwin*, London: Penguin, 1992.

De Tocqueville, A. *The Ancien Regime and the French Revolution*. London: Collins, 1966.

De Viverolles, C. *Notice biographique sur monsieur le marquis de Martainville*. Paris: Bureau central de la Revue générale, 1848.

Delabost, M. 'Un document inedit sur le Docteur Flaubert: *Notre Vieux Lycee*'. 1913.

——. *Laumonier Les Flaubert: Simple esquisse des trois surgeons de Hôtel-Dieu de Rouen pendant un siècle, 1785–1882*. Evreux: Herrisey, 1889.

Delaporte, F. *Disease and Civilisation: The Cholera in Paris, 1832*. Cambridge, MA: MIT Press, 1986.

Deleuze, M. *Histoire et description du museum royal d'histoire naturelle*. Paris: M.A. Royer, 1823.

Desan, S. 'Reconstituting the Social After the Terror: Family, Property, and the Law in Popular Politics', *Past and Present* CLXIV (1999): 81–121.

——. *Reclaiming the Sacred: Lay Religon and Popular Politics in Revolutionary France*. Ithaca, NY: Cornell University Press, 1990.

Descolin. *Description abrégée du département de l'Aube*. Troyes: F. Mallet, 1799.

Diderot, D., and J. D'Alembert (eds). *Encyclopédie, ou dictionnaire raisonné des sciences, des arts et des métiers*. Paris: chez Briasson, 1751.

Dodet, E. *Sens au XIXe siècle: L'essor de l'enseignement*. Sens: Société Archéologique de Sens, 2001.

Du Camp, M. *Souvenirs littéraires*. Paris: Hachette, 1882.

Dubois, A. 'Achille-Cléophas Flaubert', *Bulletin Flaubert–Maupassant* 15 (2004): 40–7.

Dubosc, G. 'Les Ancêtres paternels de Gustave Flaubert', *Journal de Rouen* (17 février 1924).

——. 'Un don au Musée du Pavillon Flaubert: un dessin du Dr Achille Flaubert', *Journal de Rouen* (9 aout 1922): 2.

——. *Trois Normands: Pierre Corneille, Gustave Flaubert, Guy de Maupassant; études documentaire*. Rouen: H. Defontaine, 1917.

Dubuc, A. 'Un accident ignoré du père de Flaubert', *Les Amis de Flaubert* 34 (1969): 45–6.

——. 'La bibliothèque générale du père de Gustave Flaubert' in *Les Rouennais et la famille Flaubert*. Rouen: Edition des Amis de Flaubert, 1980.

——. 'L'enterrement du père de Gustave Flaubert', *Les Amis de Flaubert* 37 (1970): 34–6.

——. 'La nomination du père de Flaubert, en 1806, à Hôtel-Dieu de Rouen', *Les Amis de Flaubert* 24 (1964): 43–6.

Dugenne, P.C. *Dictionnaire biographique, généalogique et historique du Département de l'Yonne*. Sens: Société Généalogique de l'Yonne, 2000.

Dumesnil, R. 'Comment sont morts le père et la soeur de Flaubert', *La Chronique Médicale* 29 (1922): 244–6.

Dunbar, R.G. 'The Introduction of the Practice of Vaccine into Napoleonic France', *Bulletin of the History of Medicine* 10.5 (1941): 635–50.

Dupaquier, J. *Histoire de la population française*. Paris: Presses Universitaires de France, 1988.

Elmer, P. *The Healing Arts: Health, Disease and Society in Europe, 1500–1800*. Manchester: Manchester University Press, 2004.

Entralgo, P.L. 'Sensualism and Vitalism in Bichat's "Anatomie Generale"', *Journal of the History of Medicine & Allied Science* 3 (1948): 47–64.

Fauvel, D. 'Achille-Cléophas d'après les registres de l'Hôtel-Dieu', *Bulletin Flaubert–Maupassant* 15 (2004): 59–70.

——. 'Les ancêtres champenois d'Achille-Cléophas Flaubert', *Bulletin Flaubert–Maupassant* 15 (2004): 7–12.

Fichot, C. *Album pittoresque et monumentale du Département de l'Aube*. Troyes: Imprimerie de E. Caffé, 1852.

Figlio, K. 'Review: The Birth of the Clinic', *The British Journal for the History of Science* 102 (1977): 164–7.

Finnegan, R. 'Family Myths, Memories and Interviewing' in *The Oral History Reader*, ed. R.T. Perks. London: Routledge, 2006.

Flaubert, A.-C. *Dissertation sur le manière de conduire les malades avant et après les opérations chirurgicales*. Paris: Didot Jeune, 1810.

——. 'Achille-Cléophas Flaubert to the Members of the Administrative Commission of the Rouen Hospices' (10 November 1819). Photocopy of letter, courtesy of Yvan Leclerc.

——. 'Discours de réception', pages 26–9 in *Précis analytique des travaux de l'Académie Royale des sciences, des belles-lettres et des art de Rouen pendant l'année 1815*. Rouen: P. Periaux, 1815.

——. 'Journal de Clinique' (1818), ten manuscript notebooks. Musée Flaubert et d'histoire de la médecine, Rouen.

——. 'Mémoire sur plusieurs cas de luxation dans lesquels les efforts pour la réduction ont été suivis d'accidents graves', *Répertoire générale d'anatomie et de physiologie pathologique* 3 (1827): 55–69.

—— et al. *Réponse des chefs du service de santé des hôpitaux de Rouen à un mémoire publié par MM. leurs adjoints*. Rouen: impr. de E. Periaux fils aîné, 1834.

Flaubert, G. *Œuvres complètes*, ed. B. Masson. 2 vols. Paris: Editions du Seuil, 1964.

——. *Correspondance: Volume One*, ed. Jean Bruneau. Paris: Gallimard, 1973.

——. *Correspondance: Volume Two*, ed. Jean Bruneau. Paris: Gallimard, 1980.

——. *Correspondance: Volume Three*, ed. Jean Bruneau. Paris: Gallimard, 1991.

——. *Correspondance: Volume Four*, ed. Jean Bruneau. Paris: Gallimard, 1998.

——. *Correspondance: Volume Five*, ed. Jean Bruneau and Yvan Leclerc. Paris: Gallimard, 2007.

——. *Madame Bovary*, trans. Geoffrey Wall. London: Penguin Books, 1992.

Floquet, A. 'Bordier & Jourdain', *Histoire du Parlement de Normandie: Vol VII*. Rouen: Edouard frères, 1842: 554–65.

Fontaine, J.P. *Les Mysteres de l'Yonne*. Romagnat: Editions de Borée, 2005.

Forrest, A. 'Conscription and Crime in Rural France during the Directory and Consulate' in *Beyond the Terror: Essays in French Regional and Social History, 1794–1815*, ed. G. Lewis and C. Lucas. Cambridge: Cambridge University Press, 1983.

Forster, R., and O.A. Ranum. *Medicine and Society in France: Selections from the Annales, economies, sociétés, civilisations*, volume 6. Baltimore: Johns Hopkins University Press, 1980.

Foucault, M. *The Birth of the Clinic: An Archaeology of Medical Perception*, trans. Alan Sheridan. New York: Pantheon, 1973.

Fourcroy, A. 'Première adresse des officiers du Jardin des plantes & du Cabinet d'histoire naturelle, lue à l'Assemblée nationale, le 20 Août 1790' (1790). *The French Revolution Research Collection* <http://gallica.bnf.fr/ark:/12148/bpt6k420666/f3.image> accessed 3 October 2012.

——. *Rapport et projet de décret sur l'établissement d'une école centrale de santé à Paris, fait à la Convention nationale, au nom des comités de salut public et d'instruction publique*. Paris: Imprimerie nationale, 1794.

Gay, P. *The Party of Humanity: Studies in the French Enlightenment*. London: Weidenfeld & Nicolson, 1964.

Geison, G.L. *Professions and the French State, 1700–1900*. Philadelphia: University of Pennsylvania Press, 1984.

Gelfand, M. 'A Confrontation over Clinical Instruction at the Hotel-Dieu of Paris During the French Revolution'. *Journal of the History of Medicine & Allied Science* 28.3 (1973): 268–82.

Gelfand, T. 'Gestation of the Clinic', *Medical History* 252 (1981): 169–80.

Gillispie, C. 'Chemistry, Pharmacy and Revolution in France, 1777–1809', *Medical History* 51.4 (2007): 553–5.

——. *Science and Polity in France: The Revolutionary and Napoleonic Years*. Princeton: Princeton University Press, 2004.

Gillispie, C.C. (ed.). *Dictionary of Scientific Biography*. New York: Charles Scribner's Sons, 1970–80.

Goldstein, J. *The Post-Revolutionary Self: Politics and Psyche in France, 1750–1850*. Cambridge, MA: Harvard University Press, 2005.

Goldwyn, R.M. 'Guillaume Dupuytren: His Character and Contributions', *Bulletin of the New York Academy of Medicine*. 45.8 (1969): 750–60.

Goncourt, E., and J. Goncourt. *Journal: mémoires de la vie littéraire*. Paris: Fasquelle Flammarion, 1956.

—— and J. Goncourt. *Pages from the Goncourt Journal*, ed. Robert Baldick. Oxford: Oxford University Press, 1962.

Goncourt, J. *Histoire de la societe francaise pendant la Revolution*. Paris: E. Dentu, 1854.

Gouda, F. *Poverty and Political Culture: The Rhetoric of Social Welfare in the Netherlands and France, 1815–1854*. Lanham, MD: Rowman and Littlefield, 1995.

Gregoire, H. *Histoire des sectes religieuses*. Paris: Baudoin Frères, 1828.

Grout, C.F. *Gustave Flaubert par sa nièce Caroline Franklin Grout*. Rouen: Publications de l'université de Rouen, 1999.

Gueroult, G. *Henry Barbet, Maire de Rouen 1789–1875*. Paris: Editions Christian, 2007.

Haigh, E. *Xavier Bichat and the Medical Theory of the EIghteenth Century*. London: Wellcome Institute for the History of Medicine, 1984.

Hallé, J.N. 'Hygiène moderne' in *Dictionnaire des sciences médicales*. U. S. d. M. e. d. Chirurgiens. Paris, Panckoucke. 22 HUM – HYG: 532–608. Paris: Panckoucke, 1818.

Hannaway, C., and A. La Berge. *Constructing Paris Medicine*. Amsterdam: Rodopi, 1998.

Harrison, C.E. *The Bourgeois Citizen in Nineteenth Century France*. Oxford: Oxford University Press, 1999.

Haviland, T., and L. Parrish. 'A Brief Account of the Use of Wax Models in the Study of Medicine', *Journal of the History of Medicine & Allied Science* 25.1 (1970): 52–75.

Hazareesingh, S. *The Legend of Napoleon*. London: Granta, 2004.

Hazlitt, W. *Notes of a Journey Through France and Italy*. London: Hunt and Clarke, 1826.

Hellis, D.M.P. *Clinique médicale de l'Hôtel-Dieu de Rouen*. Paris: Chez Gabon, 1826.

——. *Souvenirs du choléra en 1832*. Paris: Chez Ballière, 1833.

Henry, G. 'Les Ancêtres de la mère de Gustave Flaubert', *Les Amis de Flaubert* 47 (1975).

Hesse, C. *Publishing and Cultural Politics in Revolutionary Paris, 1789–1810*. Berkeley: University of California Press, 1991.

Heywood, C. *Childhood in Nineteenth-Century France: Work, Health and Education among the 'Classes Populaires'*. Cambridge: Cambridge University Press, 1988.

——. *Growing up in France: From the Ancien Régime to the Third Republic*. Cambridge: Cambridge University Press, 2007.

Hickey, D. *Local Hospitals in Ancien Régime France: Rationalization, Resistance, Renewal, 1530–1789.* Montreal: McGill-Queen's University Press, 1997.

Hodge, M.J.S. 'Against "Revolution" and "Evolution"'. *Journal of the History of Biology* 38.1 (2005): 101–21.

Horn, J. *The Path Not Taken.* Cambridge, MA: MIT Press, 2006.

Hossard, J. 'Le Dr Hellis: médecin de l'Hôtel-Dieu de Rouen' (1998), *Groupe d'Histoire des Hôpitaux de Rouen* <http://www3.chu-rouen.fr/NR/rdonlyres/80CEF43D-98C1-46C5-AFEF-FF4FFED5C708/0/1998.pdf> accessed 3 October 2012.

Huard, P. *Biographies Médicales et Scientifiques XVIIIe Siècle.* Paris: Roger Dacosta, 1972.

Hunt, L. *The Family Romance of the French Revolution.* Berkeley: University of California Press, 1992.

——. *Politics, Culture and Class in the French Revolution.* London: Methuen, 1984.

Jacob, M.C. *The Radical Enlightenment: Pantheists, Freemasons and Republicans.* Lafayette: Cornerstone, 1981.

Jamerey, E. *Histoire de Maizières-la-Grande-Paroisse: Arrondissement de Nogent-sur-Seine.* Paris: Livre d'histoire-Lorisse, 2004.

Jardin, A., and A.J. Tudesq. *Restoration and Reaction.* Cambridge: Cambridge University Press, 1983.

Jones, C. *The Charitable Imperative: Hospitals and Nursing in Ancien Régime and Revolutionary France.* London, Routledge, 1989.

——. *The Great Nation: France from Louis XV to Napoleon.* London: Allen Lane, 2002.

——. *The Longman Companion to the French Revolution.* London: Longman, 1988.

——. 'The Médecins du roi in the French Revolution' in *Medicine at the Courts of Europe*, ed. V. Nutton. London: Routledge, 1990.

——. 'Picking up the Pieces: The Politics and the Personnel of Social Welfare from the Convention to the Consulate' in *Beyond the Terror: Essay in French Regional and Social History 1794–1815*, ed. G. Lewis and C. Lucas. Cambridge: Cambridge University Press, 1983.

—— and R. Porter. *Reassessing Foucault.* London: Routledge, 1994.

Jones, G.S. 'An End to Poverty: The French Revolution and the Promise of a World Beyond Want', *Historical Research* 78.200 (2005): 193–207.

Jordanova, L.J. 'Has the Social History of Medicine Come of Age?', *Historical Journal* XXXVI (1993): 437–49.

Journal de l'Empire Russes à Nogent (2 mars 1814).

Kafker, F.A. 'Bourgelat, Claude' in *The Encyclopedists as Individuals: a Biographical Dictionary of the Authors of the Encyclopédie*. Oxford: Voltaire Foundation, 1988.

Kaufman, M.H. 'Wax Models', *Journal of Medical Biography* 11.4 (2003): 187.

Kennedy, M. 'The Jacobin Clubs and the Press: "Phase Two"', *French Historical Studies* 13.4 (1984): 474–99.

Klencke, H. *Lives of the Brothers Humboldt, Alexander and William*. New York: Harper and Brothers, 1854.

Kroen, S. 'Revolutionizing Religious Politics During the Restoration', *French Historical Studies* 21.1 (1998): 27–53.

Kselman, T.A. *Death and the Afterlife in Modern France*. Princeton: Princeton University Press, 1993.

Kudlick, C.J. 'Giving Is Deceiving: Cholera, Charity, and the Quest for Authority in 1832', *French Historical Studies* 18.2 (1993): 457–81.

La Berge, A. *Mission and Method: The Early Nineteenth-Century French Public Health Movement*. Cambridge: Cambridge University Press, 1992.

La Berge, A.F. 'The Paris Health Council, 1802–1848', *Bulletin of the History of Medicine* 49.3 (1975): 339.

Laumonier, J.B. *Discours sur l'anatomie*. Rouen: Boullenger, 1793.

Lavallée, J. *Voyage dans les départements de la France*. Paris: Brion, 1792.

Lebrun, F. 'Amour et mariage' in *Histoire de la population française*, ed. J. Dupaquier. Paris: Presses universitaires de France, 1988. Volume 2: 294–316.

Legrand, E. 'Review of Report from Rouen Public Health Council for 1834–35', *Revue de Rouen et de la Normandie*. Rouen: E. Legrand, 1837. Volume 11: 414.

Legrand, J. *Chronicle of the French Revolution*. London: Longman, 1989.

Leroux, J.J. *Discours prononcé sur la tombe de M. Hallé*. Paris: Imprimerie Didot le jeune, 1822.

Lesch, J.E. *Science and Medicine in France: The Emergence of Experimental Physiology 1790–1855*. Cambridge, MA: Harvard University Press, 1984.

Levasseur, L. *Les Notables de la Normandie*. Rouen: Imprimerie L. Deshayes, 1872.

Licquet, T. *Rouen, its History and Monuments, A Guide to Strangers with a Map of the Town and Five Views*. Rouen: Edward frères, 1840.

——. *Rouen, son histoire, ses monuments, ses environs*. Rouen: A. Le Brument, 1855.

Lucas, C. 'The Rules of the Game in Local Politics under the Directory', *French Historical Studies* 16.2 (1989): 345–71.

Lyon, J. 'The "Initial Discourse" to Buffon's "Histoire Naturelle": The First Complete English Translation', *Journal of the History of Biology* 9.1 (1976): 133–81.

Marc, C.H.C. 'Introduction', *Annales d'hygiène publique* 1 (1829): i–xxxix.

——. *La Vaccine soumise aux simples lumières de la raison*. Paris: J.-B. Baillière, 1836.

Marchand, J. 'L'apothicairerie de l'Hôtel Dieu de Rouen et ses apothicaires', Groupe Histoire des Hôpitaux de Rouen, Journées du Patrimoine du 14 septembre 2006 <http://www3.chu-rouen.fr/NR/rdonlyres/B1DAD9ED-C86D-4B07-A58C-5AC957015388/0/2006_marchand.pdf> accessed 3 October 2012.

Marec, Y. *Pauvreté et protection sociale aux XIXe et XXe siècles*. Rennes: Presses universitaires de Rennes, 2006.

Martin, M. 'Doctoring Beauty: The Medical Control of Women's Toilettes in France, 1750–1820', *Medical History* 49.3 (2005): 351–68.

Marx, K. *The Revolutions of 1848*. Harmondsworth: Penguin Books, 1973.

Mathiez, A. *La Théophilanthropie et le culte décadaire, 1796–1801*. Paris: Alcan, 1904.

Maulitz, R. *Morbid Appearances: The Anatomy of Pathology in the Early Nineteenth Century*. Cambridge: Cambridge University Press, 1987.

Mayne, J. *The Journal of John Mayne During a Tour on the Continent Upon its Reopening After the Fall of Napoleon, 1814*. London: John Lane, 1909.

McPhee, P. *Living the French Revolution 1789–1799*. Basingstoke: Palgrave Macmillan, 2006.

Merriman, J.M. *The Margins of City Life: Explorations on the French Urban Frontier, 1815–1851*. New York: Oxford University Press, 1991.

Michaud, L.G. 'Bichat' in *Biographie universelle ancienne et moderne*. Volume 4: Berg-Bonfrère. Paris: Mme C. Desplaces, 1843.

Mitchell, S.L. *The American Repository and Review of American Publications on Medicine, Surgery, and the Auxiliary Branches of Philosophy*. New York: Faculty of Physic of Columbia College, 1802.

Mollat, M. *Histoire des Hopitaux en France*. Toulouse: Privat, 1982.

——. *Histoire de Rouen*. Toulouse: Privat, 1979.

Murdoch, R.T. 'Newton and the French Muse', *Journal of the History of Ideas* 19.3, 323–34.

Murphy, T.D. 'The French Medical Profession's Perception of its Social Function Between 1776 and 1830', *Medical History* 23 (1979): 259–78.

——. 'Medical Knowledge and Statistical Methods in Early Nineteenth-Century France', *Medical History* 25 (1981): 301–19.

Murray, J. *A Handbook for Travellers in France*. London: J. Murray, 1854.

Noiret, C. *Mémoires d'un ouvrier rouennais*. Rouen: Brière, 1836.

Outram, D. *The Enlightenment*. Cambridge: Cambridge University Press, 2005.

———. *Georges Cuvier: Vocation, Science and Authority in Post-Revolutionary France*. Basingstoke: Palgrave Macmillan, 1984.

———. 'The Language of Natural Power: The Eloges of Georges Cuvier and the Public Language of Nineteenth Century Science', *History of Science* 16 (1978): 153–78.

Ozouf, M. *Festivals and the French Revolution*. Cambridge, MA: Harvard University Press, 1991.

Parent-Duchâtelet, D., and D'Arcet. 'De l'influence et de l'assainissement des salles de dissection', *Annales d'hygiène publique et de médecine légale* 5 (1831): 243.

Pennetier. *Le Chirurgien Laumonier*. Rouen: Imprimerie Julien Lecerf, 1887.

Perrot, P. *Fashioning the Bourgeoisie: A History of Clothing in the Nineteenth Century*. Princeton: Princeton University Press, 1994.

Petit, M.A. 'Discours sur l'influence de la Révolution française sur la santé publique' in *Essai sur la médecine du cœur*. Paris: Garnier, Reymann, 1806.

Pickstone, J.V. 'Bureaucracy, Liberalism and the Body in Post-Revolutionary France: Bichat's Physiology and the Paris School of Medicine', *History of Science* xix (1981): 115–42.

Pihan-Delaforest, A. *Premier voyage de S.A.R. Mme la duchesse de Berry en Normandie*. Paris: Pihan Delaforest, 1824.

Pinel, P. *A Treatise on Insanity*. London: Cadell and Davies, 1806.

Poitevin. *Catéchisme républicain suivi de maximes de morale propre à l'éducation des enfans de l'un et de l'autre sexe*. Paris: Millet, 1794.

Popkin, J.D. 'The Provincial Newspaper Press and Revolutionary Politics', *French Historical Studies* 18.2 (1993): 434–56.

Porter, R. *The Greatest Benefit to Mankind*. London: Harper Collins, 1997.

——— and A. Wear. *Problems and Methods in the History of Medicine*. London: Croom, 1987.

——— and W.F. Bynum. *Companion Encyclopedia of the History of Medicine*. London: Routledge, 1993.

Price, R. 'Poor Relief and Social Crisis in Mid-Nineteenth-Century France', *European History Quarterly* 13 (1983): 423–54.

Quinlan, S.M. 'Physical and Moral Regeneration after the Terror: Medical Culture, Sensibility, and Family Politics in France, 1794–1804', *Social History* 29.2 (2004).

Railliet, A.L.J., and L. Moul. *Histoire de l'Ecole d'Alfort*. Paris: Asselin et Houzeau, 1908.

Ramsey, M. *Professional and Popular Medicine in France, 1770–1830: The Social World of Medical Practice*. Cambridge: Cambridge University Press, 1988.

Ratcliffe, B.M. 'Classes laborieuses et classes dangereuses à Paris: The Chevalier Thesis Reexamined', *French Historical Studies* 17.2 (1991): 542–74.

Reibel, M. *Les Flaubert, vétérinaires champenois et l'origine de Gustave Flaubert.* Troyes: Imprimerie Gustave Fremont, 1913.

Robertson, I. *France: Blue Guide.* 4th revised edition. London: A & C Black, 1997.

Rosenberg, C.E., and J.L. Golden (eds). *Framing Disease: Studies in Cultural History.* New Brunswick: Rutgers University Press, 1992.

Rush, B. *Medical Inquiries and Observations.* Philadelphia: J. Conrad and Co., 1805.

Salgues, J.B. *La Philosophie rendue à ses premiers principes, ou cours d'études … pour servir à l'instruction de la jeunesse.* Paris: Chatain, 1801.

——. *Des erreurs et préjugés répandus dans la société.* Paris: Buisson, 1810.

——. *Troisième mémoire pour l'infortuné Lesurques.* Paris: Imprimerie de Auguste Mie, 1829.

Schiesari, J. 'Mourning and Melancholia: Tasso and the Dawn of Psychoanalysis', *Quaderni d'italianistica* XI.1 (1990): 13–26.

Schivelbusch, W. *Disenchanted Night: The Industrialization of Light in the Nineteenth Century.* Berkeley: University of California Press, 1998.

Shepherd, W. *Paris in 1802 and 1814.* 1815.

Siegfried, S.L. *The Art of Louis-Léopold Boilly: Modern Life in Napoleonic France.* New Haven: Yale University Press, 1995.

Smellie, W. 'Preface by the Translator', *Natural History General and Particular by the Count de Buffon Translated into English.* London: Strahan & Cadell, 1785.

Spary, E.C. *Utopia's Garden: French Natural History from Old Regime to Revolution.* Chicago: University of Chicago Press, 2000.

Staum, M.S. *Cabanis: Enlightenment and Medical Philosophy in the French Revolution.* Princeton: Princeton University Press, 1980.

——. 'The Class of Moral and Political Sciences, 1795–1803', *French Historical Studies* 11.3 (1980): 371–97.

Steinberg, R. 'The Afterlives of the Terror: Dealing with the Legacies of Violence in Post-Revolutionary France, 1794–1830s'. PhD thesis, University of Chicago, 2010.

Thiers, A. *Histoire de la Révolution française. Huitième édition.* Brussels: Adolphe Wahlen, 1836.

Tombs, R. *France 1814–1914.* London: Longman, 1996.

Travers, J. *Au peuple, sur le choléra-morbus par un cousin du Bonhomme Richard.* Saint-Lô: Imprimerie de J. Elie, 1831.

Veblen, T. *The Theory of the Leisure Class: An Economic Study of Institutions.* London: Allen and Unwin, 1949.

Védie, A. *Notice biographique sur M. Flaubert, chirurgien en chef de l'Hotel-Dieu de Rouen*. Rouen, Imprimerie de D. Briere, 1847.

Vernier, J.J. *Cahiers de doléances du bailliage de Troyes et du bailliage de Bar-sur-Seine pour les Etats-Généraux de 1789*. Troyes: Nouel, 1911.

Vess, D.M. *Medical Revolution in France 1789–1796*. Gainesville: University Press of Florida, 1975.

Vigné, D.M. 'Eloge de Laumonier', *Précis analytique des travaux de l'Académie des Sciences, Belles-lettres et Arts de Rouen*. Rouen: Periaux, 1819, 111–19.

Villermé, M. *Tableau de l'état physique et moral des ouvriers employés dans la manufacture de coton de laine et de soie*. Paris: Jules Renouard et cie, 1840.

Voltaire. *Philosophical Dictionary*. New York: Basic Books, 1962.

Vovelle, M. *1793 La Révolution contre l'Eglise: de la Raison à l'Etre Suprême*. Paris: Editions complexe, 1988.

Wallon, H. *Histoire du tribunal révolutionnaire de Paris*. Paris: Hachette, 1880.

Weiner, D.B. 'French Doctors Face War: 1792–1815' in *From the Ancien Régime to the Popular Front: Essays in the History of Modern France*, ed. C.K. Warner. New York: Columbia University Press, 1969: 51–73.

——. 'Public Health under Napoleon: The Conseil de Salubrité de Paris, 1802–1815'. *Clio medica Amsterdam, Netherlands* 94 (1974): 271.

——. *The Citizen-Patient in Revolutionary and Imperial Paris*. Cambridge, MA: Harvard University Press, 1993.

Weisz, T. *The Medical Mandarins: The French Academy of Medicine in the Nineteenth and Early Twentieth Centuries*. Oxford: Oxford University Press, 1995.

Williams, E.A. *The Physical and the Moral: Anthropology, Physiology, and Philosophical Medicine in France, 1750–1850*. Cambridge: Cambridge University Press, 1994.

Williams, L.P. 'Science, Education and the French Revolution'. *Isis* 44 (1953): 311–30.

Williams, R. *Marxism and Literature*. Oxford: Oxford University Press, 1977.

Woloch, I. 'Napoleonic Conscription: State Power and Civil Society'. *Past and Present* 111 (1986): 101–29.

——. *The New Regime: Transformations of the French Civic Order, 1789–1820s*. London: W.W. Norton, 1994.

Wylock, P. 'The Life and Times of Guillaume Dupuytren', *Canadian Journal of Surgery* 32.6 (1989): 4.

Young, A. *Travels in France During the Years 1787, 1788 & 1789*. Cambridge: Cambridge University Press, 1950.

Index